Can't Lose Weight?

You could have Syndrome X!

The chemical imbalance that makes you store fat!

By Dr Sandra Cabot

Can't Lose Weight?
You could have Syndrome X
Dr Cabot, Sandra

First published 2001 by WHAS
P. O. Box 54 Cobbitty NSW 2570 Australia
02 4653 1445
www.whas.com.au
www.sandracabot.com

SCB International Inc.
PO Box 5070
GLENDALE AZ 85312-5070 USA
Ph: 623 334 32 32

First Edition printed October 2001

Categories

1.Weight Control. 2. Weight Loss 3. Syndrome X. 4. Diet 5. Nutrition 6. Diabetes 7. Polycystic Ovarian Syndrome 8. Women's Health Advisory Service

Disclaimer

The suggestions, ideas and treatments described in this book must not replace the care and direct supervision of a trained health care professional. All problems and concerns regarding your health require medical supervision. If you have any pre-existing medical disorders, you must consult your own doctor before following the suggestions in this book. If you are taking any prescribed medications you should check with your own doctor before using the recommendations in this book.

Printed by Griffin Press
Typeset by Concept Factory Pty Ltd
Courtesy of "*The Rainbow Warrior*"

ISBN: 0-958-61370-2

www.sandracabot.com
www.weightcontroldoctor.com
www.liverdoctor.com

Contents

Dedication

This book is dedicated to the "unsung heroes" of the National Health Advisory Service who have worked tirelessly over the last 20 years to help people with health problems from all over the world. They are my special team without whom I would be unable to share my knowledge and inspiration. When we first started 20 years ago there was very little self-help information available on nutritional and hormonal medicine. Today the use of nutritional medicine has become main stream, but still we find that many thousands of people value and trust our Health Advisory Service. This is because they know that we are always there to help, support and advise them with knowledge and compassion.

Our phone number is 02 4655 8855.

I would also like to thank the publisher for their continuing support of Women's Refuges in Australia.

About the Author

Dr Sandra Cabot MBBS, DRCOG is a medical doctor who has extensive clinical experience in treating patients with weight problems, chronic medical problems, liver problems and hormonal imbalances. Dr Cabot works with other medical doctors and her team of naturopaths in Sydney Australia and Phoenix Arizona in the USA. Dr Sandra Cabot began studying nutritional medicine while she was a medical student and has been a pioneer in the area of holistic healing. She graduated in medicine with honours from the University of Adelaide, South Australia in 1975. During the early 1980s Dr Cabot worked as a volunteer in the largest missionary Christian hospital in Northern India, tending to the poor indigenous women.

In Australia she pilots herself to many cities and regional and country centres, where she is invited to conduct seminars and training workshops. Dr Cabot appears regularly on radio stations such as 2GB and 4BC where she is a health commentator. Her free magazine called "Ask Dr Sandra Cabot" is available through health food stores and many pharmacies. The newsletter can also be read on line at www.sandracabot.com

About Audrey Tea

The indefatigable Audrey Tea has been cooking delicious and healthy meals for well over 50 years. Born and bred in Adelaide South Australia, where Audrey's culinary talents have tantalised the taste buds of thousands, she continues to design and test recipes in collaboration with Dr Sandra Cabot. While maintaining the principles of healthy metabolism, Audrey can prepare and cook dishes, which range from fabulous family meals, gourmet dinner party menus, quick snacks, special surprises and boutique sweet treats. This skill has taken her many years to perfect and yet despite this amazing talent, she remains incredibly humble and giving.

Audrey Tea is also a recipe tester and has had to make many modifications to conventional Western recipes that we once considered healthy. Audrey helps us to discover that healthy can be gourmet and indeed is usually much tastier and satisfying than the meals that were once considered traditional Australian cuisine. She has managed to make the recipes truly multicultural, which will introduce new flavours and health benefits to you by increasing diversification of your diet.

I have been fortunate to be a recipient of Audrey's meals over the years and I hope to continue to receive her regular gifts of treats. I am now delighted to be able to share these recipes with you and your family. They come with laughter and maternal healing vibrations, just like Audrey Tea herself. Audrey Tea accompanies Dr Sandra Cabot on many of her seminar tours and is always available to answer questions on healthy cooking and menu planning.

Introduction

Greetings! My name is Dr Sandra Cabot. If you are battling with a weight problem, this book has a strategy that I truly believe can help you for the rest of your life.

I have an incredible life that has given me the opportunity to communicate face to face with hundreds of thousands of men and women. Most of these people come to see me looking for help with their weight and hormonal problems. I fly extensively, travelling thousands of miles to visit towns all over Australia that would otherwise be impossible to reach in a short time span. During my travels I will often meet around a thousand new people in a week, who relate their stories of weight problems and poor health to me. I also receive hundreds of E-mails and many letters every week from people all over the world. Some people may find this daunting but I find it fascinating and challenging. This is because I am able to offer these people a **real** and **lasting solution** to their problems. These people have tried many different things to overcome their weight problems but find that there are missing parts to the jig saw puzzle, which means that they do not know where to start. They will often relate how they have tried every possible diet on the market and taken every type of diet pill, but still continue to gain weight. They feel extremely frustrated, disappointed and confused.

The major obstacle is that they lack a plan or strategy that is tailor made for them, and takes into account **all the reasons that prevent them from losing weight**.

After 25 years of medical research and clinical practice I have been able to focus on the medical problems that prevent people from losing weight. I have also developed new treatments that can overcome these medical problems safely and naturally. They will work for you, as they scientifically attack the medical problems that cause your metabolism to be abnormal. My approach works on the **causes of weight excess**, which means that if you can adopt my program as a lifestyle, you will gradually, be successful.

If you are overweight you need to recognise the medical problems that in all probability are keeping you fat. Furthermore you need to understand how and why these problems cause you to store fat instead of burn fat. For you to be inspired to change you must understand how these changes will work in your own body.

This book is the only book that exists that takes into account ALL THE FACTORS THAT STOP YOU FROM LOSING WEIGHT. I want to have an open and honest relationship with you from the start because I am not trying to sell you a magic quick fix full of hyped up marketing. I am trying to bring back the clarity in your life, which will keep you inspired with passion to become the best you can possibly be.

> *People believe they are fat just because they eat too much, don't exercise enough or have inherited the wrong genes from their parents. This is a far too simplistic and limited attitude. Indeed these people are very surprised and often relieved to learn that they have* ***several medical problems*** *that may be making them fat.*

When a patient with a stubborn weight problem consults me, I assess them for the following medical problems –

- Do they suffer with Syndrome X?
- Do they have a dysfunctional or fatty liver?
- Do they have hormonal imbalances?
- Do they have body toxicity?
- Do they have fluid retention?
- Do they have a sluggish metabolism?
- I also assess their Body Type or Body Shape.

Only after **all the above factor**s are taken into account can they begin to use a tailor made strategy for their own individual weight problem. I think this makes a lot of sense, don't you?

I am sure you know people that seem to overeat, but manage to stay slim, and others who seem to eat very little, but remain overweight. This is because body weight is greatly affected by medical factors, and not just by how much a person eats every day. What we eat is much more important than how much we eat, because the molecules in different foods will affect our metabolism, liver function, hormones, and blood sugar control.

Do not worry that this book is going to be complicated, just because it takes into account all the factors that could be keeping you fat. This book is going to make it much easier for you to lose weight because instead of relying on one strategy only, you will have the tools to fight all the medical reasons that prevent you from achieving your goals.

To help you to be successful I have a team of dedicated people in Sydney who can support you through the phone, Internet and personal consultations in my "Dr Sandra Cabot Weight Loss Centres". I also have consultants in Perth, Brisbane, Adelaide and Melbourne.

If you need more help phone 02 4655 8855 or visit www.weightcontroldoctor.com

It can be so confusing

Twenty years ago when I started writing there was a lack of information regarding nutritional medicine and natural therapies. People were starving for information especially about natural therapies, diet and hormones. Today the opposite has happened and people suffer with information overload. Yes there are too many diets, so many supplements and so many philosophies, and in one lifetime you cannot possibly do them all! Furthermore, you cannot try all these things successfully without some form of long term support and direction.

What you need to know is what is right for you as an individual. You need to know in your particular case, if there are specific medical problems that are keeping you fat. That is why I have begun to develop a network of "Dr Sandra Cabot Weight Control Centres" where all these factors can be addressed. We are also happy to work with your own local doctor and suggest the necessary tests that your doctor may need to do. We will be holding support groups and seminars where you can share with others and gain strength from their success stories.

I recently read with amusement, an article published in a medical journal titled "Cardiologist's Fat Fight". It described the extreme clashing of expert opinions at the annual meeting of the American College of Cardiology. Supporters of the official low fat approach, argued with opponents who believed it was excess carbohydrates that caused abnormal blood fats and Syndrome X.

The main opponents were well known cardiologists Dr Robert Atkins, and Dr Dean Ornish who had totally opposite views on the best diet to prevent Syndrome X and its leading complication of cardiovascular disease.

Dr Atkins promoted his low-carbohydrate, high-fat, high-protein diet, while Dr Ornish promoted a rigorous vegetarian diet low in fat and high in complex carbohydrates. If the experts have totally different approaches and cannot agree, then who can?

I believe that the types of food we eat on a regular basis are crucial to our health and weight control success, and in most of my patients I need to make dietary changes. I find that it is extremely rare to find someone who has a "perfect diet", especially bearing in mind that this means different things to different people, including the experts!

It is true that when we look around, people are generally eating less fat and more carbohydrates, and yet they are getting fatter! Indeed some experts believe that a high carbohydrate, low-fat diet can be dangerous to your health and lead to obesity and diabetes.

But I have also found that it is **not the diet alone** that needs to be considered, but the other individual medical problems that may be sabotaging even your best efforts at following a "healthy diet", no matter whose diet you follow. Yes we need to look a little deeper into our health in much the same way as a detective would solve a mysterious case. Let us find the missing pieces to the jig saw puzzle so that we can see the overall picture and begin the holistic approach that leaves no stone unturned. Only then are our chances of success very high.

The missing parts to the jig saw puzzle are –

- Syndrome X
- The state of your liver
- Hormonal imbalances
- Sluggish metabolism
- Body toxicity
- Your Body Type

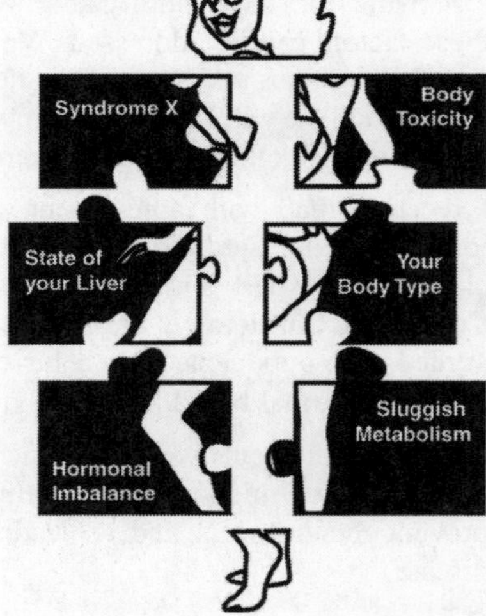

So stay with me and allow me to help you solve the puzzle. Read on and discover that what seems at first to be hidden and mysterious, is in fact obvious and simple to overcome. We need a combination of nutritional and modern day medicine to beat the epidemic of weight excess and degenerative disease that threatens most developed countries.

An interesting case history

During one of my seminars in 1999, I met a woman who really showed me how important it is to consider all the medical reasons that can make a person chronically obese and unwell. Donna was 47 years old and had suffered with polycystic ovaries for many years, which unfortunately had been inadequately treated. Donna was very overweight, and being an Android Body Type (apple shaped) she carried all of her excess weight in her upper body and abdomen. She had lost most of her hair and was almost bald in the male pattern of baldness, although she hid this well with a coloured headband over her forehead. She had a fatty liver, Syndrome X and was hypertensive. Although she was almost of menopausal age, she complained of heavy menstrual bleeding, which was due to the deficiency of the hormone progesterone, commonly seen in women who do not ovulate regularly. She was taking the drug "Aldactone", in an attempt to reduce her excessive male hormones but this was not controlling her hormonal and metabolic imbalance. Indeed she was going nowhere and had been trapped in a hormonal and metabolic nightmare for years. I thought to myself "if only I had been able to see this woman 20 years ago, what a difference I could have made to her physical and mental state". This woman needed specific help to address ALL of the medical problems that were making her fat and destroying her looks. However it is never too late to restore normal body chemistry and she was still looking for a solution after all these years.

I started her on my dietary program for Syndrome X, and gave her supplements to reduce her high insulin levels and reduce her cravings for carbohydrates. I also stopped the Aldactone, which was not helping her bleeding and hair loss. I prescribed the anti-male hormone called "Androcur", which acts as a type of progesterone to reduce heavy bleeding, and is also very effective at reducing high levels of male hormones.

To be able to balance her metabolism and get her excess weight off, I had to –

- Reverse the chemical imbalance of Syndrome X
- Balance her hormones
- Improve her liver function
- Take into account her Body Type

Someone like this presents a real challenge, and needs powerful strategies that look at ALL the imbalances that perpetuate obesity.

Within 6 months I had brought her hormonal problems under control, so that her bleeding had gone and her hair was growing back. Lowering the male hormones had made it much easier for her to lose the weight from her upper body, as excess male hormones increase insulin resistance and thus fat gain.

It took me 2 years to reverse her fatty liver condition and during this time, as her liver started to burn fat normally, she gradually lost her abdominal obesity. The supplements and liver tonics had also helped her to speed up her sluggish metabolism.

It gave me great satisfaction to see this woman change from an obese masculine balding woman, to an attractive middle aged woman with thicker hair and a normal body weight.

1

Chapter One

What is Syndrome X?

What has your weight got to do with insulin?

The hormone insulin is made in the pancreas gland, and is secreted into the blood stream by the gland in response to a rise in blood sugar (glucose). After circulating in the blood stream for only 6 to 10 minutes, the insulin binds with specific receptors on the cell membranes to transfer glucose from the blood stream inside the cells. The hormone insulin is extremely powerful and controls the processing of blood sugar.

Everything you eat and drink is absorbed from the small intestine and passes into the portal vein, which takes the nutrients from the meal straight to the liver. Fats are broken down into glycerol and fatty acids, while protein is broken down into amino acids, and all these travel to the liver for processing. Carbohydrates are absorbed from the gut as simple sugars, which quickly become glucose.

Insulin attaching to the cell receptor

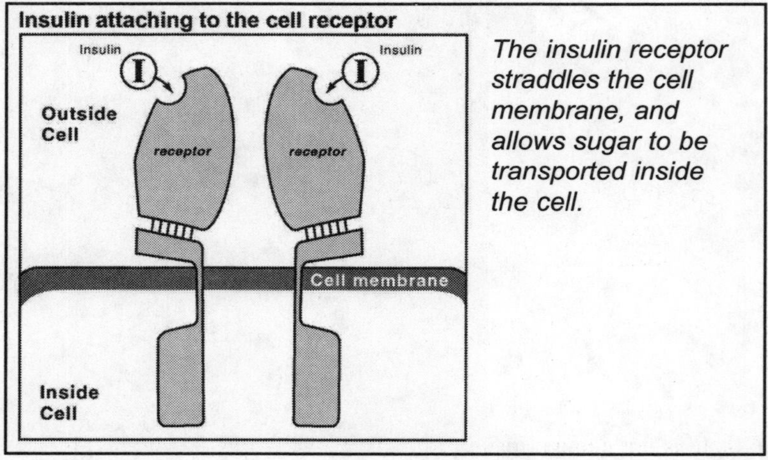

The insulin receptor straddles the cell membrane, and allows sugar to be transported inside the cell.

If you eat a lot of carbohydrate this will produce a lot of glucose in your blood stream. Glucose is pure energy, and your body has to decide how much of this glucose it will use for immediate energy needs, and how much glucose it will store for future energy needs. It is the powerful hormone insulin, which makes this decision and sends the glucose to the areas of your body that are most suitable and accessible. After a meal, as the blood glucose rises the pancreas pumps out insulin, which converts some of the blood glucose into a starch called glycogen, which is stored in the muscle and liver cells for future use. Once the glycogen stores are full, excess blood glucose will be converted by the insulin into fat, which is called triglyceride. This triglyceride can be carried in your blood stream to the fatty tissues where it will be deposited as more fat. So we could say that insulin encourages the storage of fat, and that is why **insulin has been called "the fat- producing hormone**".

Body Glands and their Hormones

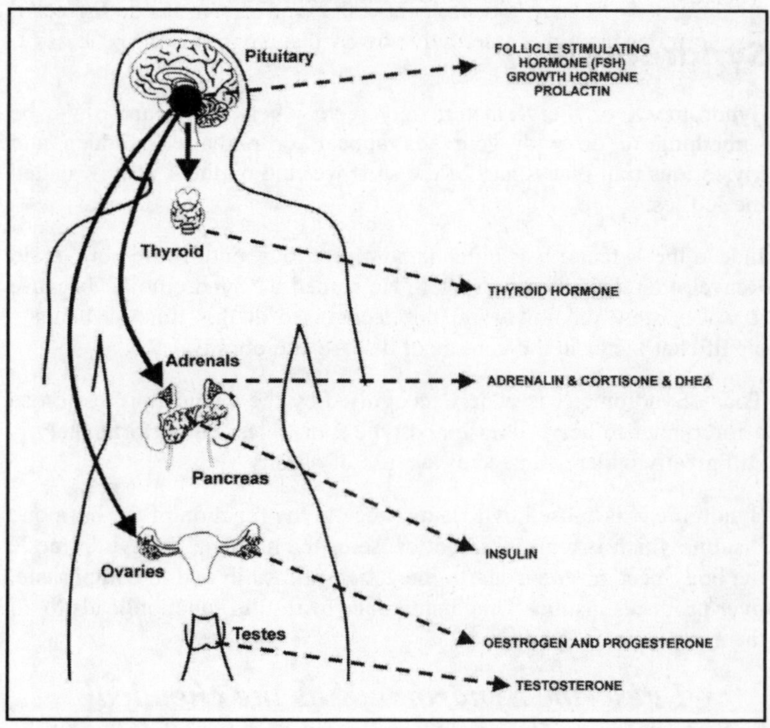

If there is not enough insulin as in type 1 diabetics, the blood glucose is not transferred into glycogen or fat, and the levels of blood glucose rise to dangerously high levels. If there is too much insulin, the blood glucose drops to dangerously low levels so that there is not enough to fuel the brain. This sends emergency signals to your hormonal system, which responds by pumping out hormones such as adrenalin, cortisol and glucagon to liberate glucose urgently into the blood stream.

The types of foods in your diet will have a big effect upon the amount of insulin that you have in your blood stream. If you eat meals that are high in refined carbohydrates, such as white flour and sugar, the blood glucose will rise rapidly causing a rapid increase in insulin levels. Meals containing mostly fat and protein, but low in carbohydrates, do not cause a large rise in blood glucose, and therefore do not require much insulin to be processed. Protein foods require a little insulin, whereas fat requires virtually no insulin to process.

Syndrome X

Syndrome X or the X factor, may seem when first heard of, to be something to do with your sex appeal, or perhaps a hidden and mysterious trait that is part of the stuff we find on the TV show called the X-files.

Indeed the X factor was hidden and mysterious, until Professor Gerald Reaven first described it in 1988. He named it "Syndrome X" because it was largely unknown and not recognised at this time as being a significant factor in the genesis of disease and obesity.

Today Syndrome X is widely recognised by the medical profession as a forerunner to heart disease and type 2 diabetes, but unfortunately is still greatly underestimated as a cause of obesity.

Syndrome X is caused by a disturbance in the function of the hormone insulin, which is really the root cause of the problem. In Syndrome X the body becomes resistant to the action of insulin and to compensate, over produces insulin. This disturbance of insulin function leads to all the symptoms of Syndrome X.

I describe Syndrome X as the chemical imbalance that makes you fat. Syndrome X is the most powerful medical reason why people cannot lose weight. Indeed Syndrome X makes it virtually impossible to lose weight unless it is specifically treated.

What is Syndrome X?

It is a collection of symptoms and medical signs that we find in one patient. These include –

- **Insulin resistance**
- **High levels of the hormone insulin**
- **Abnormalities in blood fats**
- **A variety of blood sugar abnormalities**
- **There may also be high blood levels of the acid called uric acid.**
- **High blood pressure may be present**
- **Weight excess especially in the abdominal area**

Professor Reaven's research team first recognised that people with insulin resistance and high blood levels of the hormone insulin have an elevated risk of heart disease. Reaven also found that a high carbohydrate diet could raise the insulin levels and thus the risk of heart disease. Professor Reaven called Syndrome X the "metabolic syndrome" which is seen in people who are insulin resistant. Although Syndrome X is usually associated with weight excess, it can also be found in non-obese, non-diabetic persons.

Let us now look at these individual signs that collectively form Syndrome X

Insulin Resistance

This term means that the body is resistant to the effects of the hormone insulin, so that your body has lost the ability to respond to the insulin. Your body cells resist the insulin so that the pancreas has to secrete more insulin to make up for this lack of sensitivity. In those with insulin resistance the insulin is not able to transfer glucose from the blood into the cells very efficiently. This causes the blood glucose levels to rise.

The resistance to insulin results from defects in the sensitivity of the body cells to insulin. The body cells become insensitive to insulin because the receptors on the surface of the cells do not communicate efficiently with the insulin.

It is as if the receptors become accustomed to the high insulin levels and become desensitised to them – it's like the boy who cried wolf and in the end no one took him seriously.

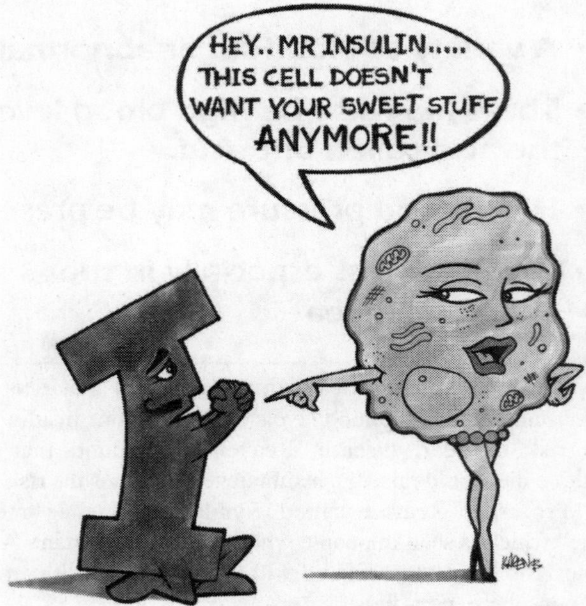
HEY.. MR INSULIN.....
THIS CELL DOESN'T
WANT YOUR SWEET STUFF
ANYMORE!!

Yes the snobby cells just ignore the insulin!

What causes Insulin Resistance (IR) ?

In modern day industrialised societies around 1/3 to 1/2 of the population is unable to metabolise carbohydrates efficiently. This is due to a combination of genetics, excess carbohydrate intake and a lack of exercise.

Weight excess can cause insulin resistance, and resistance to the action of insulin is a characteristic feature of human obesity. It is the ingestion of too much refined carbohydrate that triggers the release of high levels of insulin, but the body cells cannot respond to this insulin. Because the insulin does not work efficiently, the pancreas responds by pumping out even more insulin to try to overcome this resistance. In insulin resistance (IR) the insulin becomes less and less effective at converting glucose into cellular energy, and more of this glucose is transferred into fat deposits. Therefore we find that high levels of insulin, and IR occur in the vast majority of overweight people.

In those with IR, although the insulin cannot get glucose into the cells efficiently, it can still perform other functions such as converting carbohydrates into fat and suppressing the burning of stored fat. In a normal person, around 40% of dietary carbohydrate is converted into fat, whereas in a person with IR, that percentage is often much higher. People with IR are not designed to eat large amounts or even moderate amounts of carbohydrates.

In people with normal insulin metabolism the body cells are **not** resistant to the action of insulin and only small amounts of insulin are required to control the blood sugar levels. These people do not battle with their weight, as excess quantities of the fat producing hormone insulin are not produced. Their blood sugar levels are generally more stable, so that they do not get the strong cravings for carbohydrates so typical of those with IR. These people are designed to be able to eat more carbohydrates without metabolic problems.

In those with IR, symptoms such as fatigue, mental fogginess, mood changes, shakiness and insatiable hunger for carbohydrates frequently occur. This is because the glucose is not getting inside the cells so that the cells are not producing adequate energy. Thus you don't have the energy to exercise, which makes it harder to lose the weight.

In IR, there may also be a delayed responsiveness of your cells to insulin, so that at first the high amounts of insulin do not work. Eventually some hours after eating, the insulin starts to work, causing a large drop in blood sugar, so you suffer with hypoglycaemia. Hypoglycaemia makes you extremely tired and unable to function mentally or physically. This causes a sudden urge to eat more carbohydrates, which then send up the insulin levels again, so that the glucose is converted to fat. Yes, you feel trapped in a vicious cycle believing that it is your will power that is at fault. Well, stop feeling guilty, because you are a victim of a chemical imbalance and not a weak personality.

You are locked into a metabolic problem that is making you fatter and fatter!

If this chemical imbalance is allowed to continue it could result in diabetes. Diabetes occurs when the cells are so resistant to insulin, that the blood sugar continues to rise to abnormally high levels and remains continuously elevated. Diabetes is extremely common in overweight people and there are now approximately one million Australians who have diagnosed diabetes. Eventually the insulin may fail completely and weight loss will then begin because there is not enough insulin to transfer the blood glucose into glycogen or body fat. The pancreas becomes totally exhausted and is unable to keep on producing the huge amount of insulin that is required to control the blood sugar levels. This is called pancreatic burnout and it is then necessary to prescribe insulin therapy.

High levels of the hormone insulin

In Syndrome X the blood insulin levels become elevated because the body needs higher and higher amounts of insulin to control the blood glucose levels.

High levels of insulin are damaging to your health for several reasons:

- They cause the blood fat called triglyceride to become elevated.
- They cause the good cholesterol (HDL) levels to go down.
- They cause the liver to manufacture more of the bad (LDL) cholesterol.
- They increase the development of fatty plaques in your arteries (atherosclerosis).
- They increase the retention of salt and water and stimulate the growth of smooth muscle cells in the arteries, which elevates blood pressure.
- They may affect the brain chemicals (neuro-transmitters), causing mood disorders and insomnia.
- They stimulate hunger, especially for high carbohydrate foods.
- They promote the transfer of blood glucose into triglyceride fats and thus encourage fat deposits in your body – **in other words insulin tends to make you fat.**

- They **suppress** the levels of two important slimming hormones in your body –
    - Glucagon - which promotes the burning of sugar and fat.
    - Growth hormone - which is needed for building new muscle mass.

You can see that **high levels of insulin increase the risk factors for cardiovascular disease**. Because obesity and high insulin levels usually go together explains why being overweight is a major risk factor for your heart. If we can stop the vicious cycle of insulin resistance and high insulin levels, you will not only have a powerful weapon to lose weight, you will also be able to reduce your risk of heart disease and increase your life span.

Abnormalities in blood fats

These include the following –

» Cholesterol abnormalities

Elevated insulin levels stimulate your cells to produce abnormally large amounts of cholesterol. In those with Syndrome X there will be low levels of the good HDL cholesterol, and excessively high levels of the bad LDL cholesterol.

Let's talk about cholesterol, which is generally a poorly understood subject. Around 80% of the body's cholesterol is made in the liver and the cells of the small intestine, and only around 20% comes from the diet. If you eat more cholesterol your liver will make less, so a healthy liver is vital for maintaining a healthy cholesterol balance.

Cholesterol is a waxy pearly like fat and is not soluble in watery fluids such as the blood stream. To carry cholesterol around in your blood stream it must be coated with protein. Protein coated cholesterol particles are called lipoproteins. The amount of protein coating the cholesterol determines how dense it is – the higher the protein content the higher the density will be.

Around 20% of your blood lipoproteins are high-density lipoproteins, which we abbreviate to HDL. HDL is beneficial because it scavenges cholesterol from your cells and arteries and carries it back to the liver.

The liver recycles and processes the cholesterol, and can pump excess amounts out of the body through the bile. Thus we can say that the liver is a "fat burning" and a "fat pumping" machine.

Around 65% of the blood lipoproteins are low-density lipoprotein, which we abbreviate to LDL. LDL is known as the "bad cholesterol" because it carries cholesterol to your cells and blood vessels.

HDL is protective against cardiovascular disease, so **you want your HDL levels to be as high as possible**. Contrary to popular belief, desirable high levels of HDL cholesterol are not achieved with a low-fat diet. What we find is that HDL is often undesirably lowered by a low – fat, high - carbohydrate diet. Reducing refined carbohydrates and eating the good fats (essential fatty acids) will increase the levels of the good HDL cholesterol.

Normal levels of HDL are (1.0 to 1.9) mmol/L in men and (1.2 to 2.3) mmol/L in women

Normal levels of LDL are (0.5 to 3.5) mmol/L

Lipoprotein (a)
Lipoprotein (a) abbreviated to Lp(a), is a sticky form of LDL cholesterol, which can increase the risk of clots and blockages in your blood vessels. High levels of Lp(a) are a potent risk factor for heart disease.

The normal Lp(a) range is (0 to 270) mg/L.

Abnormally high levels of Lp(a) can be partly hereditary, and are also affected by your diet. It is known that eating large quantities of hydrogenated and partially hydrogenated fats (the transfatty acids), can elevate Lp(a) levels undesirably. These undesirable fats are found in most margarines and many processed and packaged foods. You can reverse this by eating plenty of salads and vegetables, seeds, nuts and legumes. A reasonable amount of unprocessed saturated dietary fat as found in eggs, seafood, coconut and fresh lean meats will also help to lower Lp(a)

» High levels of blood triglycerides

Triglycerides are lightweight small fatty particles that have only a very small amount of protein attached to them. Most of the triglycerides are stored as fat in your fat deposits, and a small amount is sent to the muscle cells for energy. The triglyceride fats are manufactured in the liver, which converts them to very low-density lipoproteins abbreviated to VLDL. High levels of triglycerides and VLDL will not only increase weight gain, they will increase your risk of cardiovascular disease.

Those with Syndrome X have a build up of "triglyceride – rich – lipoproteins" (fatty protein particles) in the blood after eating. High blood levels of insulin cause the liver to produce very low-density lipoprotein triglyceride (VLDL-TG). This is very dangerous and predisposes to fatty liver, atherosclerosis, and obesity.

Today many people have become obsessed with cholesterol and think it is the main predictor of heart disease. Indeed many overweight people never bother to have their triglyceride levels checked, often because their doctor does not think it is important. This is dangerous neglect, because high triglyceride levels by themselves, irrespective of cholesterol levels, are a potent risk factor for heart disease. Indeed high triglyceride levels are just as important as smoking, obesity and high blood pressure in increasing your chances of heart disease. High triglycerides make your blood thick and sticky so that it does not flow freely around inside your blood vessels – this increases the risk of blood clots.

Normal triglyceride levels are = (0.5 to 2.0) mmol/L, and the lower they are within this normal range the better off you are.

The **combination of high triglycerides and low HDL cholesterol is very dangerous for your heart,** and is more predictive of heart disease than any other ratio. *(REF. 2)*

Make sure that you are fasting (do not eat/drink anything but water for 12 to 14 hours before the blood test), when you have your blood taken to measure the triglyceride levels. This is because triglyceride levels can be temporarily much higher just after eating.

It is relieving to know that changing what you eat, exercising a little and taking some supplements is able to reverse this deadly combination within a few months, and sometimes sooner. And you will not have to follow a low-fat, low-calorie diet to do this, so you will not be hungry or miserable. A study at Harvard University in 1966, showed that very high triglyceride levels could be reduced greatly with a very low carbohydrate diet *(REF. 3)*

A diet high in refined carbohydrates (those with a high glycaemic index), and low in protein and fat, will cause secretion of high levels of insulin, which will cause an elevation in the triglyceride levels. *(REF. 4)*

Conversely a diet low in carbohydrates, and particularly low in refined carbohydrates, will lower elevated triglycerides and raise low levels of the desirable HDL cholesterol. Of course it is important to improve the function of the liver, which is the organ most concerned with regulation of fat metabolism. To improve liver function you need to increase your consumption of raw and cooked vegetables and take a good liver tonic.

A variety of blood sugar abnormalities

In those with Syndrome X the ***blood sugar levels are often unstable, and can vary from too low to too high.*** As the disease progresses, the blood sugar levels generally become too high.

In type 2 diabetics the blood sugar level stays above normal because they do not have enough insulin to transfer sugar from the blood into the cells.

In contrast, in those with Syndrome X, the pancreas responds by secreting extra insulin to overcome the insulin resistance, and blood sugar levels remain lower than diabetic levels. Syndrome X can however eventually lead to type 2 diabetes, as the insulin resistance gets worse, causing blood glucose levels to rise.

In Syndrome X there may be wide fluctuations in the levels of blood glucose from too high to too low. Abnormally high levels of blood glucose are known as hyperglycaemia, and abnormally low levels of blood glucose are known as hypoglycaemia. Hyper means "too much", and hypo means "too little".

Hypoglycaemia

When the blood sugar levels drop below 2.5 to 3 mmol/L, the following symptoms may occur –

- **Strong cravings** for refined carbohydrates such as sugar, sweet drinks, chocolate, bread or even alcohol.
- **Emotional changes** such as anxiety, poor concentration, "foggy brain", poor memory, irritability, depression and rapid mood changes.
  The anxiety may be associated with shaking, sweating,

palpitations and panic attacks. This is due to the body's response to levels of glucose that are too low to supply the needs of the brain. This sends signals to the glands to pump out hormones such as adrenalin, glucagon, and cortisol to rapidly raise the blood sugar levels. This is vital to protect the brain's supply of glucose, but these hormones can cause the anxiety, sweating, shaking and palpitations that are so unpleasant.

- **Sleep disturbances**, such as waking suddenly from sleep with anxiety and palpitations, bad dreams, and restless sleep.
- **Mental and physical fatigue** which can be overwhelming, and tends to occur in between meals and especially in the midafternoon.

Hypoglycaemic symptoms can be devastating, and it is not uncommon to find sufferers who think they are battling with a mental illness. Anti-depressant drugs will not help these symptoms, as they do not correct the underlying unstable blood sugar levels. Many people with depression and addictions can be helped with an eating program and supplements to stabilise their blood sugar levels. The sugar addiction can become so strong that you feel totally out of control until you can get your sugar hit.

One of my patients called Mandy, had an interesting presentation of hypoglycaemia. She was a 26-year-old mother of two, and experienced panic attacks and a weight increase during the week before her menstrual bleeding. She would yell at the children, feel very tired and could not cope with any stress at all. She found her solace in chocolate, which temporarily took away her symptoms. I decided to do two tests on Mandy at day 21 of her menstrual cycle, which is approximately 7 days before the onset of menstrual bleeding. I measured her progesterone levels and did a 3-hour glucose tolerance (GTT) test.

I was not surprised to discover that she had very low levels of the hormone progesterone and severe hypoglycaemia. During the GTT, she experienced a panic attack when the blood sugar (glucose) reached its lowest level. In Mandy's case, her low levels of progesterone plus her high dietary sugar intake were causing the hypoglycaemia. I treated Mandy with natural progesterone lozenges and increased her consumption of regular protein and essential fatty acids, and her next cycle was "just a breeze" as she said. "I was not even aware that it was that time of the month, and I could cope with normal life and the children", she explained to me on her follow up visit.

Yes, it is not only diet that can affect our blood sugar levels but hormones as well. This is why it is important to balance the hormones in women with hypoglycaemia, that occurs pre-menstrually and during the peri-menopausal years, and also in women with post-natal depression. Because sex hormones are steroid hormones, they can help to reduce hypoglycaemia in women with hormonal imbalances. Natural oestrogen, progesterone and testosterone may all help in hormonally triggered hypoglycaemia.

Other chemical imbalances of Syndrome X

The high levels of insulin suppress the action of the fat burning hormone called glucagon.

There may be high blood levels of the acid called uric acid, which increases the risk of gout and kidney disease.

There may be high levels of "plasminogen activator – 1" in the blood, which means the ability to break up blood clots is reduced. This increases the risk of heart attacks and strokes.

High Blood Pressure

As many as 50 percent of people with high blood pressure (hypertension), have the chemical imbalance of Syndrome X reflected in insulin resistance and high levels of insulin. High insulin levels cause retention of sodium and water by the kidneys, and increase the pressure inside the peripheral smaller blood vessels. These things will elevate the blood pressure.

Abdominal obesity

If you carry excess body fat in the abdominal area, and find it very difficult to lose the weight there is a very high chance that you have Syndrome X. Insulin has a much stronger effect upon fat cells in the abdominal area, and high levels of insulin will cause fat storage most easily in the abdomen and upper body. Abdominal obesity is associated with high levels of insulin, and therefore with all the other risks of high insulin, such as abnormal blood fats, high blood pressure and a predilection to heart disease and diabetes.

Where you carry your excess body fat is even more important for your health than your total weight. If you store excess weight in the abdominal area it is important to understand where this excess fat is laid down. The excess fat not only accumulates underneath the skin of the abdominal wall, but also inside the abdominal cavity and around your body organs. In the early stages, the fat accumulates around the liver, stomach, pancreas, intestines and kidneys. As Syndrome X progresses, the increasing fat begins to accumulate around the heart, and starts to infiltrate or invade the body organs, so you may develop a fatty pancreas, fatty kidneys, or worst of all a fatty liver.

Abdominal obesity is more common in men and in Android (apple-shaped) women, but can eventually occur in anyone with Syndrome X, if fat accumulation continues unabated.

High levels of insulin can promote storage of excess fat anywhere in the body. However if you carry most of your excess fat around your buttocks, hips and thighs, and not around your abdomen, you will be less likely to develop the higher risk of heart disease and diabetes that comes with abdominal obesity. This is because in the hip and thigh areas, there are no body cavities or vital organs that can be infiltrated with fat. The excess fat accumulates only in the layers between the muscles and skin, and often produces a marbled or cellulite appearance to the surface of the buttocks, hips and thighs. If the pear shaped (gynaeoid) woman continues to gain body fat, her excess fat may eventually accumulate in the abdominal area, and she will become a victim of Syndrome X. It is not uncommon to find that pear shaped women who have carried excess weight in the thigh/hip area for years, without any metabolic problems, suddenly put on a lot of weight in the abdominal area during the peri-menopausal years. They will then find it very difficult to shift the weight as they are beginning to develop the chemical imbalance of Syndrome X.

How common is Syndrome X?

Syndrome X is very common, and may be seen in as many as one in four persons, or 25% of a normal non-diabetic population. *(REF. 1)*

In Australia over 4 million people have Syndrome X.

In the USA approximately 60 million people have the chemical imbalance of Syndrome X.

In the USA there are approximately 16 million people with type 2 diabetes, which suggests that one in four people with Syndrome X eventually become diabetic.

2

Chapter Two

What causes Syndrome X?

What Causes Syndrome X?

Incorrect diet

The statement that "it is not how much you eat, but what you eat that's important", has never been more true than in the genesis of Syndrome X.

In this day and age the food keeps getting faster and faster, and we are getting slower and slower!

The consumption of refined carbohydrates containing white sugar and flour, has produced the epidemic of Syndrome X we have in the developed world today.

We have evolved for hundreds of thousands of years, subsisting on a cave man's diet of meat, fish and vegetables and fruits – in other words totally unprocessed and low in refined carbohydrates.

Heart attacks were not common at the start of the twentieth century, and in 1930, heart attacks caused only 3000 deaths in the United States. *(REF. 5)*

When we take a look at the diets of people who lived in the early 1900s, we find that the amount of fat in the daily diet was generally higher than it is today, when we are in the midst of an epidemic of obesity. The main types of fats eaten by those who lived in the early 1900s were butter, lard and tallow. According to modern day medical opinion, the consumption of such fats should have produced an epidemic of heart attacks and obesity, but it did not.

They did not eat the trans-fatty acids that bulk up the processed foods we eat today.

In the early 1900s, the types of carbohydrates consumed were not refined, and consisted of unprocessed grains and cereals, unrefined flour and unrefined molasses. They did eat sugar, but not in the refined packaged and fast foods that we now find lining the supermarket shelves.

Today it is not uncommon for Australians to eat nearly half a kilogram of white sugar, high fructose corn syrup and refined grains every day. We also eat large amounts of partially hydrogenated vegetable oils that contain trans-fatty acids. Trans-fatty acids are completely unnatural and are widely found in the modern Australian diet, so that they have replaced the natural essential fatty acids. It is the consumption of trans-fatty acids, as well as excessive amounts of refined carbohydrates, that have caused Australians to become fatter over the last century.

Weight Excess

Syndrome X is more common in those whose excessive weight accumulates in the upper body. This means the excess fat is found in the abdominal area and the trunk. The rest of the body may be quite muscular and relatively free of fat. Thus Syndrome X is more common in those with the Android Body Type, also known as the apple shaped body type – *see page 166.* However any Body Type that becomes overweight can develop Syndrome X.

The fat may form rolls or spare tyres around the chest, abdomen and upper hips. These are sometimes called "handle bars", and there are those who cheekily call them "love handles"!

Interestingly, upper level body fat produces more male hormones such as androstenedione, and it is known that high levels of male hormones can increase insulin resistance.

If you are overweight and you lose weight you will become less insulin-resistant. The good news is that you do not need to lose massive amounts of weight to reduce Syndrome X, and the typical over-weight individual can significantly reduce insulin resistance by losing only 8 to 10 kilograms.

Polycystic Ovarian Syndrome

Polycystic Ovarian Syndrome (PCO) is a very common hormonal imbalance in women, affecting 6 to 10% of pre-menopausal women. PCO Syndrome often leads to an excess production of male hormones. The term Polycystic Ovarian Syndrome is derived from the presence of small fluid filled sacs or cysts which accumulate in the ovaries from trapped eggs, which were never released from the ovaries. This is because normal ovulation or release of the eggs at the middle of the menstrual cycle is inhibited. Because ovulation does not occur very often, these women do not produce adequate amounts of the hormone progesterone. This results in infertility and very infrequent menstrual bleeding. This lack of progesterone can also result in heavy irregular menstrual bleeding. Women with PCO Syndrome usually have higher levels of male hormones or androgens, which are produced in their ovaries, adrenal glands and also in their upper level body fat. Weight excess will aggravate the hormonal imbalances of PCO Syndrome, and is often associated with Syndrome X. The excess of male hormones will increase insulin resistance so that blood sugar problems, high cholesterol, and hypertension may result, especially in overweight women.

Women with PCO Syndrome have a much higher risk of Syndrome X and a sevenfold increased risk of becoming a type 2 diabetic, especially if they are overweight.

Although insulin-sensitising medications such as Metformin can help those with PCO Syndrome, dietary changes remain the best strategy for long term success. Some women with PCO Syndrome are treated with the oral contraceptive pill, which produces a regular menstrual bleed. However long term use of the contraceptive pill, especially pills containing masculine progesterones, may aggravate insulin resistance and weight gain in some women with PCO Syndrome.

PCO Syndrome can often be controlled very well with weight loss, and the use of natural progesterone and nutritional supplements. Natural progesterone is given in the form of lozenges or creams, in a dose of 100 to 400mg daily for 2 weeks in every month. Natural progesterone does not aggravate insulin resistance or increase weight, and may help to relieve many symptoms of PCO Syndrome. You need a doctor's prescription for natural progesterone. Useful supplements for women with PCO Syndrome are phyto-estrogen capsules or powder, and liver tonics, which help the liver to metabolise the excessive levels of male hormones. Women with PCO Syndrome should eat only organic poultry and meats free of growth promoting hormones. They will also benefit from the eating plan in this book.

Genetic factors

Genetic factors are important in assessing your risk of Syndrome X. If you have a family history of obesity, diabetes type 2, hypertension, polycystic ovaries or heart disease, your risk of Syndrome X will be higher.

Fitness and exercise

Insulin resistance is far more common in those who have a sedentary lifestyle and do not exercise regularly. Lack of fitness may increase your risk of Syndrome X by 20 to 25%. Although exercise reduces insulin-resistance, this benefit is lost if you stop exercising.

Smoking may aggravate insulin resistance slightly, whereas 1 to 2 drinks of alcohol per day, do not seem to increase the tendency to the chemical imbalances of Syndrome X

Medications

The chemical imbalance of Syndrome X can be accelerated by some drugs such as diuretics, the oral contraceptive pill, steroids such as body building hormones or cortisone, or alcohol.

As you can see, there are several factors that can play a role in the genesis of Syndrome X, which gives a researcher a profound respect for the complexity of this disorder. Although Syndrome X is complex, we now know how to overcome it. We do this with new nutritional strategies that make some of the previously so-called "healthy conventional diets" somewhat obsolete and ineffective. You may not be surprised by this statement, as I am sure that many of you will have found that conventional low-calorie, low-fat, high-carbohydrate diets did not work for you.

Why is Syndrome X still largely unknown?

Whenever I give a public seminar and ask the audience who has heard of Syndrome X, only one or two people out of several hundred will raise their arm. Syndrome X is not recognised widely because there is a tendency to focus on, and treat the symptoms of this chemical imbalance, rather than attack the cause.

The cause of Syndrome X is a disturbance of insulin metabolism resulting in insulin resistance and excess levels of insulin.

Some researchers have compared Syndrome X to an iceberg with its cause hidden beneath the surface of the ocean. At the top of the iceberg we see only the peaks of ice, which represent the symptoms. The symptoms we see are obesity, abnormal blood fats, high blood pressure, and disturbances of blood sugar levels. Doctors treat these symptoms with drugs to lower cholesterol and triglycerides, drugs to lower blood pressure and drugs to lower blood sugar. These drugs may be needed but hopefully not forever, if we are able to attack the insulin disturbance, which is the cause of these symptoms. Excess body fat is a symptom of Syndrome X, and is usually treated with a low-fat high-carbohydrate diet. However this type of diet does not lower the raised insulin levels and insulin resistance, which is the cause of the obesity. We need an eating plan and supplement program that will normalise the insulin metabolism. Only then are we able to overcome the obesity, and all the other symptoms of Syndrome X at the same time.

Syndrome X is still not recognised as the huge threat to longevity and health that it really is. When evaluating the risks for heart attacks and atherosclerosis, the most deadly combination is high triglycerides and low HDL cholesterol. High levels of insulin and insulin resistance cause high triglycerides and low HDL cholesterol. These are the abnormalities we find in those with Syndrome X, so obviously it should be getting more attention. Not only is Syndrome X the leading medical cause of obesity, it is also a leading cause of cardiovascular disease.

The Iceberg of Syndrome X

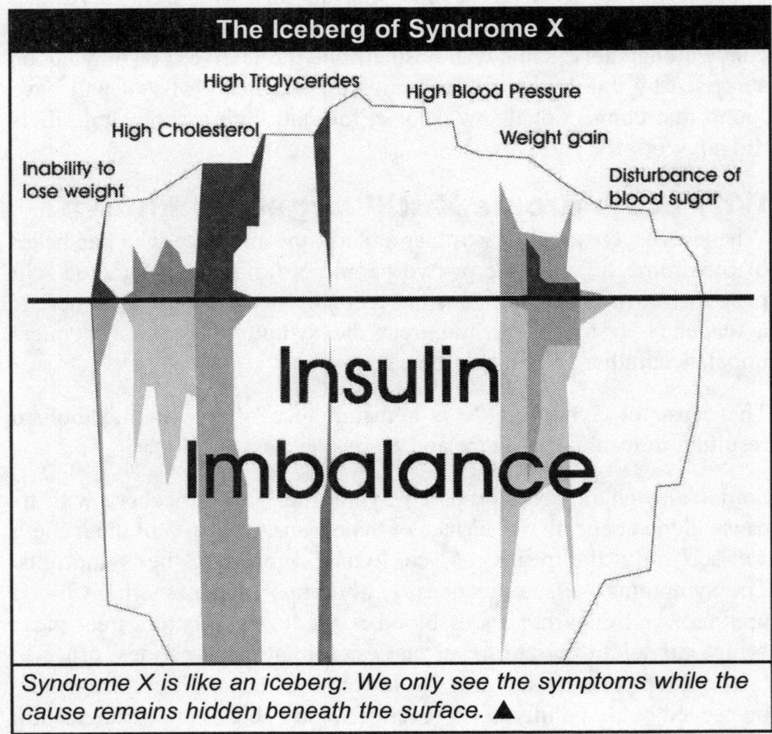

Syndrome X is like an iceberg. We only see the symptoms while the cause remains hidden beneath the surface. ▲

3

Chapter Three

How do we diagnose Syndrome X?

How do we diagnose Syndrome X?

Your own doctor may be interested in doing laboratory tests to see if you have Syndrome X.

You will need to have your blood taken in the fasting state, which means that you should not eat/drink anything apart from pure water, for 12 to 14 hours before the blood is taken. It is easiest to fast overnight and have your blood taken before breakfast.

Tests to evaluate your degree of Syndrome X –

- **Fasting levels of the blood fats**

Fats	Normal range (in mmol/L)
Total cholesterol	3.9 to 4.5 (under 20 years of age)
Total cholesterol	3.9 to 5.5 (over 20 years of age)
Triglycerides	0.1 to 2.0
LDL cholesterol	0.5 to 3.5
HDL cholesterol	1.0 to 1.9 (males)
HDL cholesterol	1.2 to 2.3 (females)

The Ratio of $\frac{\text{total cholesterol}}{\text{HDL}}$ is predictive of your risk of heart disease as follows —

Chol/HDL ratio	RISK OF HEART DISEASE
2.5 to 3.5	below average (desirable)
3.6 to 5.5	average
5.6 to 8.3	high
> 8.3	very high

• Fasting Blood Sugar Level (BSL)

If your fasting BSL is over 6.1 mmol/L, this means that insulin is starting to lose its control over your blood sugar levels. This is a sign of insulin resistance.

• Glucose Tolerance Test

The Glucose Tolerance Test (GTT) measures the tolerance of an individual for an extra load of administered glucose. If your tolerance for this extra load of glucose is normal, then your blood levels of glucose will remain within the normal range. If your tolerance for this extra load of glucose is impaired, your blood sugar levels will become higher than the normal range *(see table 1 - pg-42)*.

If you have impaired glucose tolerance, this will be because you have insulin resistance, meaning that your insulin is incapable of controlling your blood sugar levels. If your blood sugar levels become even higher you will be classed as a diabetic, which could be due to severe insulin resistance or insulin failure.

The GTT will only be accurate if you follow a relatively high carbohydrate diet (200 grams daily) for four days before the test.

The GTT measures your blood sugar (glucose) levels after you ingest a test dose of glucose. The blood sugar levels are measured over a period of several hours, depending on whether the doctor has ordered a 2-hour GTT, or a GTT which goes for longer. A five-hour GTT is much more revealing in those with Syndrome X, or disturbances of blood sugar control.

You may be asked to fill out a questionnaire of your symptoms during the period of the GTT, with the aim of matching your symptoms to the reading of your blood sugar level. Symptoms such as faintness, shaking, sweating, palpitations, nausea, mood changes, mental confusion and extreme hunger are suggestive of very low blood sugar levels, or an abnormally rapid drop in the blood sugar levels. Even if you are not asked to fill out a questionnaire, it is a good idea to keep a record of your symptoms and their timing during the GTT. This may help your doctor to interpret the significance of your blood sugar levels, to the way you feel day to day.

Subtle abnormalities in the GTT often occur in those with Syndrome X, a long time before the onset of diabetes.

Blood Sugar Levels (in mmol/L) during the GTT

Time	Normal	Impaired Glucose Tolerance	Diabetes
Fasting	3.6 to 6.1	6.1 to 6.9	over 6.9
2- hour	< 7.1	7.2 to 11.0	over 11

TABLE 1

The one-hour blood glucose level is not always reported, but generally speaking a level over 9.0 mmol/L is considered abnormal, and is indicative of impaired glucose tolerance.

Ideally insulin levels should be tested along with the blood glucose levels, at least for the first 2 hours of the GTT. The fasting level of insulin should be checked, as well as the insulin level 2 hours after the patient ingests the glucose. The accepted normal value for the 2-hour level of insulin varies between the experts because insulin testing is still in its early stages. According to some experts the 2-hour insulin level is abnormally elevated if it is 1.5 times your age, up to the age of 50. Using this method a 2-hour insulin level of 75 would be abnormally high for any person.

• Serum Insulin Levels

It is a worthwhile endeavour to measure insulin levels, as it is the high insulin levels and insulin resistance, which are the cause of Syndrome X.

A laboratory accustomed to measuring insulin levels should do the testing of your insulin levels. The specimen of blood should be frozen and the test must be completed within 24 hours of taking the blood. If these procedures are not followed the results may be inaccurate.

Excessive blood levels of insulin (hyperinsulinaemia) are diagnosed by finding an elevated fasting blood insulin level, or by finding an elevated insulin level two hours after giving the patient a 75-gram dose of pure sugar (glucose).

Many research laboratories use the fasting normal levels of insulin in healthy young people as the standard reference against which we measure a patient's blood insulin levels. Generally speaking if your fasting insulin level is over 10 mU/ml, you probably have some degree of Syndrome X, meaning that you are developing insulin resistance. The greater your insulin level is over 10, the greater is your insulin resistance. If we use 10 as the upper limit of normal for fasting insulin levels, a result of 30 would mean that it requires 3 times the normal amount of insulin to keep your blood sugar levels at their current value. Some laboratories will set the upper limit of normal fasting insulin levels as high as 25 to 30, but this may miss some people with insulin resistance, who have not yet lost control of blood sugar levels. The measurement of insulin levels during a Glucose Tolerance Test (GTT) is subject to wide inter – and intra - individual variation, which can cause some difficulty with interpretation.

However normal insulin levels during a GTT are considered to be the following –

Time	Normal Serum Insulin (in uU/ml or mu/L)
Fasting	less than 11 (many labs will report anything below 20 as normal)
1 hour	9 to 60
2 hour	5 to 50
3 hour	1 to 24

TABLE 2

Some laboratories have different "normal ranges" for serum insulin, which are higher than the above values, and may miss some people with Syndrome X. For example some laboratories will state that insulin levels below 70 are normal, while insulin levels above 80 indicate insulin resistance. They qualify this by saying that insulin levels between 70 to 80 are in a "grey area" and may indicate insulin resistance. I think the lower levels in table 2 are more realistic, and if used for evaluation, will not miss as many people who are in the early stages of Syndrome X.

Because of the wide variation in insulin levels during a GTT, most endocrinologists evaluate the fasting insulin level only, and if this is not raised a diagnosis of insulin resistance is thought to be unlikely. Usually insulin resistance is inferred if there is impairment of glucose tolerance.

• Glycosylated haemoglobin levels

Glycosylated haemoglobin levels can be abbreviated to Hgb A1 or GHB. They are sometimes also abbreviated to HbA1c, which is helpful to know if you are looking at your own blood test results.

The measurement of Hgb A1 levels evaluates the amount of sugar that has been present in your blood over the previous 3 months. The Hgb A1 actually measures the amount of blood sugar that is bound to the pigment in the red blood cells. This pigment is known as haemoglobin. The higher the blood sugar levels are, the greater the amount of sugar bound to haemoglobin will be. Higher levels of Hgb A 1 will reflect this. Red blood cells remain in the blood circulation for an average of 90 days, so the levels of Hgb A 1 will reflect the average blood sugar levels over the previous 3 months. Thus the lower your level of Hgb A 1 is, the better you will be, as far as blood sugar control is concerned. The normal laboratory range for Hgb A 1 is (4 to 6%).

In type 2 diabetics good blood sugar control is present when the Hgb A1 is less than 7%. Diabetics who keep their Hgb A1 levels close to or below 7%, have a much better chance of preventing diabetic complications, such as diseases affecting the eyes, kidneys and nerves, compared to those diabetics whose Hgb A1 levels are 9% or greater.

The United Kingdom Prospective Diabetes Study (UKPDS) demonstrated the importance of reducing Hgb A 1 levels. This study showed that every percentage point decrease in Hgb A 1, reduces the risk of:

Vascular complications by	35%
Heart attacks by	18%
Diabetes related death by	25%

You should aim for your Hgb A 1 level to be at the lower limit of the normal range, and certainly not towards the upper limit. If your Hgb A 1 level is above the normal range you are certainly suffering with the insulin resistance of Syndrome X, and indeed may be pre-diabetic or even diabetic. It is important to know your level of Hgb A1, as it reflects your blood sugar levels over the previous 3 months.

• Uric acid levels

Uric acid levels are often elevated in those with Syndrome X, and this increases the risk of kidney disease and gout. The more insulin-resistant you are, the more likely it is that your uric acid levels will be on the high side. It has also been found that heart attack victims tend to have higher blood levels of uric acid.

Normal blood levels of uric acid are –

NORMAL URIC ACID LEVELS (in mmol/L)	
Males	0.2 to 0.4 (blood levels)
Females	0.1 to 0.3 (blood levels)
Urine Levels	1.8 to 40 per 24 hours (in a 24 hour collection sample of urine)

• Liver Function tests

It is not uncommon to find that the blood levels of liver enzymes are slightly elevated in those with Syndrome X, especially if they are carrying excess weight in the abdominal area. This is usually associated with some degree of fatty liver. The infiltration of unhealthy fat into the liver causes some inflammation of the liver cells. Liver enzymes become elevated when the liver is inflamed.

LIVER TESTS	NORMAL RANGES
Total Bilirubin	3 to 18 umol/L
Liver Enzymes (see below)	
AST	5 to 45 U/L
ALT	5 to 45 U/L
AP	30 to 120 U/L
GT	5 to 35 U/L

• Sex hormone levels

High levels of insulin tend to increase the blood levels of testosterone, and reduce the levels of the protein called Sex Hormone Binding Globulin (SHBG). This results in raised levels of the free androgens (male hormones) in the blood. The free androgens are unbound to the SHBG, and are thus far more active. High levels of free androgens increase the tendency to weight gain in the upper part of the body.

The normal range for free androgens is measured as the Free Androgen Index (FAI) and is –

SEX	FAI normal range
Males	40 to 170
Females	0.1 to 7

Why are high blood levels of sugar dangerous?

Sugar or glucose is sticky, which is evident when you get sugary substances stuck on your fingers. When there are large amounts of glucose circulating around in your blood stream, the glucose sticks itself onto many of your body's proteins. This process is called glycosylation. This is not a good thing as glycosylation of proteins changes the chemical structure of the proteins, causing them to bind together or cross-link with each other. The researcher who first discovered the glycosylation phenomena in living tissue was Anthony Cerami. He named the proteins damaged by sugar binding to them, "Advanced Glycosylation End-products", abbreviated to AGE's.

When sugar attaches to protein, it damages the protein in a way that can be described as cooking your proteins – similar to cooking meat. If the proteins are damaged they cannot perform their functions efficiently, and many health problems can start to arise.

Glucose can damage the many thousands of proteins that your body needs to function well. Proteins including haemoglobin, albumin, lipoproteins, enzymes, membrane proteins and collagen can be damaged by glucose.

When collagen is damaged by AGE's it loses its flexibility, so that your tissues, joints and organs are not well supported – in other words your skin starts to age more rapidly. When the proteins in the lens of your eyes are damaged by glucose, the lens becomes murky and cataracts start to form. This is a common complication of diabetes.

The protein haemoglobin is found inside your red blood cells and carries oxygen to the cells around your body. Glucose can easily attach itself to the haemoglobin protein and damage it, which affects the oxygenation of your tissues. This can slow down metabolism increasing the tendency to weight gain.

When the glucose attaches to haemoglobin it is called "glycosylated haemoglobin", abbreviated to HgbA1. Doctors often measure the amount of HgbA1 in your blood to check how much sugar your proteins are carrying. Indeed this test of HgbA1 is commonly done in diabetics, and gives us a good idea of the average levels of blood sugar over the previous 3 months.

Probably the most worrying aspect of glycosylation of proteins is that this process can occur to the proteins present in your brain cells. In the brains of Alzheimer's patients, we find tangles, plaques and deposits of dead tissue called amyloid. These abnormal structures can arise from dead cells whose proteins have been damaged by glycosylation. AGE's have been found to be present in excessive amounts in the plaques of brains affected by Alzheimer's disease. Thus it is thought that impaired glucose metabolism is important as a risk factor for Alzheimer's dementia. *(REF. 6)*

AGE's can also attach themselves to the lipoproteins such as LDL cholesterol, which makes it much harder for the LDL cholesterol to be removed from the blood circulation. This also explains why those with Syndrome X have high levels of LDL cholesterol, which will increase the risk of heart disease.

The AGE's will damage many of the important proteins in your body, which accelerates the onset of degenerative diseases and the ageing process.

So although sugar is sweet, it does not have such a sweet effect in your body when it is consumed in excessive amounts.

4

Chapter Four

Triple strategy to overcome Syndrome X

Triple strategy to overcome Syndrome X

1. Reduce high insulin levels
2. Help insulin to work better
3. Improve your liver function

All the above will facilitate weight loss

1. Reduce Insulin Levels

To lower insulin levels, we need to lower blood sugar levels and keep them stable so preventing wild fluctuations of blood sugar. If the blood sugar is persistently high the pancreas will pump out high and sustained amounts of insulin thus elevating blood insulin levels. If the blood sugar becomes excessively low, this causes the release of other hormones such as adrenalin and cortisol from the adrenal glands. These hormones cause the blood sugar to rise rapidly, which will then stimulate the pancreas to pump out excess levels of insulin so that the blood sugar levels fall again. Thus the blood sugar levels go up and down precipitously, causing extreme cravings for sugar and carbohydrates and sometimes for alcohol. These cravings are very powerful, so that the sufferer becomes addicted to sugary foods and is unable to stay away from these problem foods.

My eating plan will stabilise the blood sugar levels, thus reducing the blood sugar highs and lows. This prevents the very high levels of insulin and other hormones such as adrenalin and cortisol. High levels of adrenalin and cortisol can elevate the blood pressure, cause anxiety, headaches, tremors and sweating. High levels of the hormone insulin make you very hungry so that you need larger amounts of food to feel satisfied. Some people with Syndrome X feel so hungry they could eat the door off the refrigerator!

Eating plan summary

• Reduce refined carbohydrates

The most important carbohydrates to reduce are those that are refined and made from white sugar and white flour. Refined carbohydrates are those with a high Glycaemic Index (GI). The Glycemic Index (GI) is a standard scale used to measure the ability of specific carbohydrate foods to elevate blood sugar levels. Pure glucose (white sugar) is used as the standard measure of the GI and is given the number of 100 on the GI scale. Foods with a lower GI have a lower number on the scale. For example lentils and beans are much lower on the GI scale than bread and sweets, while meat, eggs, seafood and poultry are virtually zero. *See page 116* for more information on the Glycaemic Index.

Foods that have a high GI number are typically refined or simple carbohydrates, and will cause elevation of blood sugar and insulin levels, especially if they are eaten alone without protein or fat.

Refined carbohydrates are found in many highly processed breads, many packaged cereals, sweet cakes, biscuits and cookies, chips, pastry, some types of pasta, candies, lollies, chocolate, ice-cream, and packaged snack foods.

Overeating carbohydrates can prevent a higher percentage of fats from being used for energy, which leads to an increase in fat storage. Your body has a limited ability to store excess carbohydrates, and it will convert these excess carbohydrates into body fat.

There are many versions of the popular high protein/low carbohydrate diet, and their carbohydrate content varies considerably. I recommend around 40% of your daily calories, come from complex carbohydrates. In general, your carbohydrate intake should be roughly equal to your protein intake. As you progress with weight loss, you can gradually increase carbohydrates to approximately 10% more than your protein intake.

The tolerance to carbohydrates varies greatly between individuals, from 60 grams daily to 300 grams daily. This depends upon body weight, amount of exercise, and insulin metabolism, and some experimentation may be needed to determine what is best for you.

Refined carbohydrates should ideally be eliminated. Refined carbohydrates stimulate the production of insulin much more than complex carbohydrates do. If the carbohydrates are complex they contain fibre and nutrients, which will slow down the rapid rise in blood glucose and insulin levels.

By limiting carbohydrate intake, we can increase fat burning to provide an efficient source of energy.

• Eat first class protein with every meal

First class protein suitable for Syndrome X is found in the following food groups –

- All seafood – such as fish, shellfish, squid, octopus
- Poultry (free range is best)
- Meats – red and white (must be very fresh and lean)
- Eggs (boiled, poached, scrambled, or omelette)
- Protein powder (whey protein has the highest protein content) *see page 216*

Combination of any 3, from the following 4 groups – legumes (beans, lentils, peas) with grains with nuts with seeds. If you do not eat 3 of these 4 groups at the SAME TIME, you will not be getting all of the essential amino acids at one meal.

By eating carbohydrates with some fat and protein at the same meal, we are able to reduce the rapid insulin-stimulating rise in blood sugar.

Refined carbohydrate foods stimulate the secretion of the fat producing hormone insulin, whereas non-carbohydrate foods – fats and proteins do not stimulate the production of insulin.

• Eat some raw plant food with every meal

This includes all raw fruits and vegetables. A maximum of 3 pieces of fruit daily is allowed if you are overweight. An unlimited amount of green vegetables is allowed. Raw food increases fibre, improves digestion, and provides the best source of antioxidants. The consumption of raw food with every meal is vital in Syndrome X, as raw foods contain living vitamins and enzymes to revitalise the impaired metabolism. By eating more vegetables you will reduce your total consumption of fat and calories, and lower blood sugar and insulin levels. This will increase your chances of a longer life.

2. Help insulin to work better

It is possible to help the body to respond better to the effects of insulin. We can achieve this by improving the sensitivity of the body cells to insulin, and by preventing excessively high levels of blood sugar. By doing this we will reduce the need for the pancreas to produce excess amounts of insulin, which will assist weight loss.

There are specific herbs and nutrients that have been proven to improve glucose and insulin metabolism. They may be taken individually or combined together in some formulas for a synergistic effect.

The most effective are a combination of the following-

• Gymnema Sylvestre (GS)

According to several human clinical trials the action of the herb Gymnema Sylvestre can be beneficial in those with elevated blood sugar levels. High blood levels of glucose (hyperglycaemia), high cholesterol and excessive glycosylation of proteins, which are associated with insulin resistance, appear to be corrected by Gymnema Sylvestre. It is postulated that the beneficial action of GS works by regenerating damaged beta cells in the pancreas. The beta cells produce insulin and are often damaged in diabetics. Gymnema also reduces cravings for sugar and refined carbohydrates.

Clinical trials of Gymnema Sylvestre used an equivalent of 400mg daily of the whole herb from a 5:1 extract of Gymnema Sylvestre. *(REF. 7)*

• Bitter Melon

The herb Bitter Melon is also known as Momordica Charantia, or bitter gourd.

The fruit of this plant, which is a member of the Cucurbitaceae family, is a popular food in India. Clinical trials and laboratory experiments using an extract of the dried fruit or ground seeds of Bitter Melon, revealed its ability to lower blood sugar levels. These studies found that Bitter Melon is an effective hypoglycaemic agent that reduces excessive blood sugar levels and improves glucose tolerance in Type 2 diabetics. Although its exact mechanism of action has not been fully explained, Bitter Melon is a proven hypoglycaemic agent. In other words, it is able to reduce blood sugar levels, thus reducing the need for high insulin output.

The recommended daily dosage of Bitter Melon is an equivalent of 5 grams of the fruit powder using an 8:1 standardised extract. *(REF. 8)*

• Chromium picolinate

Chromium is required for the healthy function of the insulin receptors, which are situated on the surface of the cells. This is very important for those with insulin resistance where the receptors malfunction, and become resistant to the action of insulin. In other words chromium helps the cells to communicate better with the insulin hormone, thereby facilitating the transfer of glucose from the blood stream inside the cell to be used as cellular energy. Deficiency of chromium is common in those who have consumed a diet high in refined carbohydrates. In those with Syndrome X, I highly recommend a supplement, which contains chromium picolinate, along with synergistic factors, to make the chromium more efficient. It is difficult to get all the chromium you need from your diet, as the richest sources are Brewer's yeast and liver.

Chromium is a vital component of Glucose Tolerance Factor (GTF) which improves insulin function. Those who are deficient in chromium have difficulty in regulating blood sugar levels. Chromium deficiency may be associated with anxiety, fatigue, sugar cravings, excess hunger, glucose intolerance and high cholesterol. Many people who supplement with chromium picolinate find that their craving for carbohydrates and sweets diminishes greatly. There have also been reports that chromium supplements can help the conversion of excess fat into lean muscle tissue.

Chromium picolinate has been shown to reduce insulin resistance, lower blood sugar levels by 18%, and glycosylated haemoglobin (HgbA1c) by 10%. *(REF. 9 & 10)*

Chromium picolinate is a bioactive source of this essential mineral. The efficiency of chromium absorption is very low, but the picolinic acid in the Chromium Picolinate form is a mineral transporter, which transports chromium into the muscle. Chromium picolinate is an excellent supplement for sports people and diabetics.

Results from a study in Beijing by Anderson et al., indicate that chromium may be efficacious in treating type 2 diabetes. The metabolic effects of chromium picolinate in this large study of type 2 diabetics were comparable to oral hypoglycaemic agents or insulin.

A randomised study in 1996 of 180 patients with type 2 diabetes, showed that chromium picolinate improved blood glucose and insulin levels, cholesterol and glycosylated haemoglobin.

• Lipoic Acid

Lipoic acid is a natural substance, which has been demonstrated to be effective in improving glucose utilisation and reducing the glycosylation of proteins, both of which are critical to managing those with Syndrome X or diabetes. Improving the utilisation of glucose will contribute a great deal towards preventing the complications of diabetes such as hypertension, kidney disease, heart disease, cataracts, and neuro-degenerative disorders. Ageing is associated with free radical damage and glucose intolerance, and lipoic acid can slow this destructive process down. Lipoic acid participates in the oxidative decarboxylation of pyruvate, which places it at the crux of the conversion of glucose into energy.

Lipoic acid has repeatedly been shown to counteract insulin resistance in muscle tissue, and this is the major mechanism whereby it effectively lowers blood sugar levels. The potent antioxidant action of lipoic acid may be very useful in slowing the development of diabetic cataracts and neuropathy. Supplementation with lipoic acid provides substantial health benefits to those with Syndrome X, and also to both type 1 and 2 diabetics. Doses of lipoic acid range from 100 to 600mg daily.

(REF. 11)

• Carnitine fumarate

Carnitine is a natural substance made in the human body from the essential amino acids lysine and methionine. It is well established that carnitine is essential for the maintenance of good health in humans.

Carnitine is involved in fat mobilisation, and when it is deficient, overweight persons often find it very difficult to get into the fat burning area of metabolism. In other words, they have difficulty beginning the breakdown of body fat, which is called the stage of lipolysis and ketosis. Carnitine can be described as the "shovel" that puts the fuel into the energy factories (mitochondria) inside the cells to be converted to energy. Carnitine transfers fatty acids across the mitochondrial membrane to be used as fuel. It may help to clear the accumulation of fatty acids from the blood, which can be a problem in those with impaired glucose tolerance. Carnitine is involved in the utilisation of ketone bodies for energy, and ketones are often elevated in those on very low carbohydrate diets or in poorly controlled diabetics.

It has been reported that supplemental carnitine can reduce total blood fats, especially triglycerides. Carnitine deficiencies may contribute to potentially dangerous elevations in triglycerides and cholesterol. *(REF. 12)*

Supplemental carnitine may increase the burn rate of calories from stored fat by enhancing the efficiency of fatty acid oxidation. The richest dietary sources of carnitine are red meats (lamb and beef). Vegetables, fruits and many cereals contain little or no carnitine.

• Selenium

Selenium should be supplemented in those with Syndrome X, and in diabetics, because of its proven protective effects on cell membranes and genetic material. Selenium is the vital partner for glutathione to exert its antioxidant effects. *(REF. 13)*

• Synergistic Minerals

Magnesium, manganese and zinc are involved in multiple enzyme systems within the energy producing mitochondria. A diet high in carbohydrates, especially of the refined types, may cause depletion of trace minerals such as manganese, selenium and zinc, which will have an adverse effect upon the immune system, and slow down metabolism. Magnesium has been shown to reduce insulin resistance and I highly recommend that you take supplemental magnesium. Trace mineral deficiencies are not uncommon in those with Syndrome X, and may worsen glucose intolerance. *(REF. 14)*

The nutrients discussed above are helpful for -

- Insulin resistance and insulin excess (hyperinsulinaemia) = Syndrome X
- Unstable blood sugar levels including high blood sugar levels (hyperglycaemia) and low blood sugar levels (hypoglycaemia)
- Cravings for sugar and high GI carbohydrates
- Weight excess in those with impaired glucose tolerance

Precautions while using natural supplements

Insulin dependent diabetics must not stop their insulin medication. Diabetics on oral hypoglycaemic drugs can only stop their medication with their own doctor's approval.

Those taking the above supplements for the first time may notice that their blood sugar levels drop excessively, and this can be avoided by eating at least 3 regular meals daily, with every meal containing first class protein. Healthy in between meal snacks may also be required, consisting of nuts, seeds, sardines, tuna, crabmeat, salads or protein powder.

These nutrients will not interact adversely with insulin or oral hypoglycaemic drugs.

The patient must be guided by his/her own doctor.

Suitable doses are shown below and need to be taken 2 or 3 times daily with meals.

- Gymnema Sylvestre (5:1 standardised extract) 27.0mg equiv. to 133.3mg
- Bitter melon (8:1 standardised extract) 208.3mg equiv. to 1666.7mg
- Chromium picolinate 134mcg
- Lipoic acid 70mg
- Carnitine fumarate 150mg
- Selenomethionine 8.6mcg
- Magnesium aspartate 16.7mg
- Manganese chelate 3.3mg
- Zinc chelate 1.33mg
- Vitamin E 20i.u.

For more information on Syndrome X you may call the Health Advisory Service on 02 4655 8855

Other nutrients to reduce Insulin Resistance

To increase the sensitivity of your cells to insulin you need to –

- Improve the quality of your cell membranes
- Improve the function of the receptors on the cell membranes, which attach to the insulin molecule.

We have already discussed how the mineral complex chromium picolinate can improve the function of the insulin – receptor communication.

Another way to increase the sensitivity of your cell membrane receptors to insulin is to ensure that your diet contains abundant **essential fatty acids** of the omega 6 and omega 3 variety. These essential fatty acids can be supplemented by taking cold pressed flaxseed oil in a dose of one tablespoon daily, and also by grinding whole flaxseeds in a coffee grinder into a fine powder. You can add one tablespoon of this powder to your cereal, smoothies or desserts, to provide extra omega 3 essential fatty acids.

You should also eat plenty of oily fish such as salmon, sardines and tuna, which also provide first class protein as well as omega 3 fatty acids.

I also recommend that you eat raw nuts and seeds regularly as these are high in essential oils. Supplements of evening primrose oil, blackcurrant seed oil and borage oil, will further boost your intake of the essential omega-6 fatty acids. Capsules containing a combination of Flaxseed oil, evening primrose oil and lecithin can also be very useful in boosting the intake of both omega 3 and omega 6 essential fatty acids.

The mineral **magnesium** can have a beneficial effect upon the sensitivity of the cell membranes to insulin, which means that magnesium supplements may reduce insulin resistance. A low magnesium level has been associated with relative insulin resistance, high levels of insulin and blood sugar abnormalities.

3. Improve your liver function

Surprisingly, most people with weight excess do not think it has much to do with their liver. Indeed we mostly think about the liver as an organ to filter the toxins out of the blood stream and make vital proteins for our body. Doctors are not taught at medical school that liver function has anything to do with weight control, and doctors generally only focus on the liver if it becomes diseased. However we need to think about the liver as a very strategic organ in our plan for weight control. The healthy liver regulates fat metabolism, and is the major fat burning organ in the body. The liver makes the good HDL cholesterol, which goes out into the circulation like a little warrior and scavenges the bad LDL cholesterol, and carries it back to the liver for processing and recycling. The liver is also able to pump excess and unwanted fat out of the body via the bile, so it is carried out of the body in the bowel actions.

Fatty liver

Many overweight people have a fatty liver, which is not burning fat efficiently. A fatty liver does the opposite of what it is programmed to do, and stores fat, becoming a warehouse for fat. Obviously a fatty liver is not able to burn fat efficiently, which makes it very difficult for you to lose weight.

A healthy liver is really just a big filter with many spaces containing blood. The blood in the liver spaces is circulating from the gut via the liver, back to the right side of the heart. The spaces are separated by rows of liver cells called hepatocytes. These specialised liver cells remove the excess fat from the blood in the spaces and process it. If however your liver is fatty, the liver cells are full of fat, and cannot remove enough fat from the blood in the spaces. Thus the blood remains full of fatty particles, which circulate around the body and deposit in your fatty areas. The liver cells become choked with the unhealthy fat accumulated within them. This fat takes up space within the liver cells, so that the fat squashes the tiny organs within the cells. We could say that your liver cells become obese. Such obese cells are unable to manufacture the good HDL cholesterol and vital proteins, so that your metabolism slows down, and your cholesterol levels become elevated.

In a fatty liver we could say that the liver cells are being invaded by unhealthy fat. The fat is acting somewhat like a "cancer", and is replacing the healthy liver cells with fat.

Because fatty liver is so common, it used not to be considered as a liver disease. However this attitude is changing, as we now know that fatty infiltration of the liver can impair liver function, cause liver inflammation, and may lead to cirrhosis of the liver. In severe cases of fatty liver a liver transplant may be required.

How to tell if you have a fatty liver

You will have the following problems –

- Accumulation of fat in the abdominal area
- There may be a roll of fat around the upper abdomen – I call this the "liver roll" – *see diagram page 66*
- Inability to lose weight
- You may have abnormal blood fats – high LDL cholesterol and triglycerides, and low HDL cholesterol
- You may have high blood pressure
- An ultrasound scan of the liver will show that the liver has an abnormal texture with fatty infiltrations and streaks of fat.
- Your liver enzymes may be elevated if the fat is causing liver inflammation. In the early stages your liver enzymes may not be elevated. This can be tested for with a simple blood test.

The condition of fatty liver is also known in medical terms as Non-Alcoholic Steatorrhoeic Hepatosis (NASH) or steato-hepatitis.

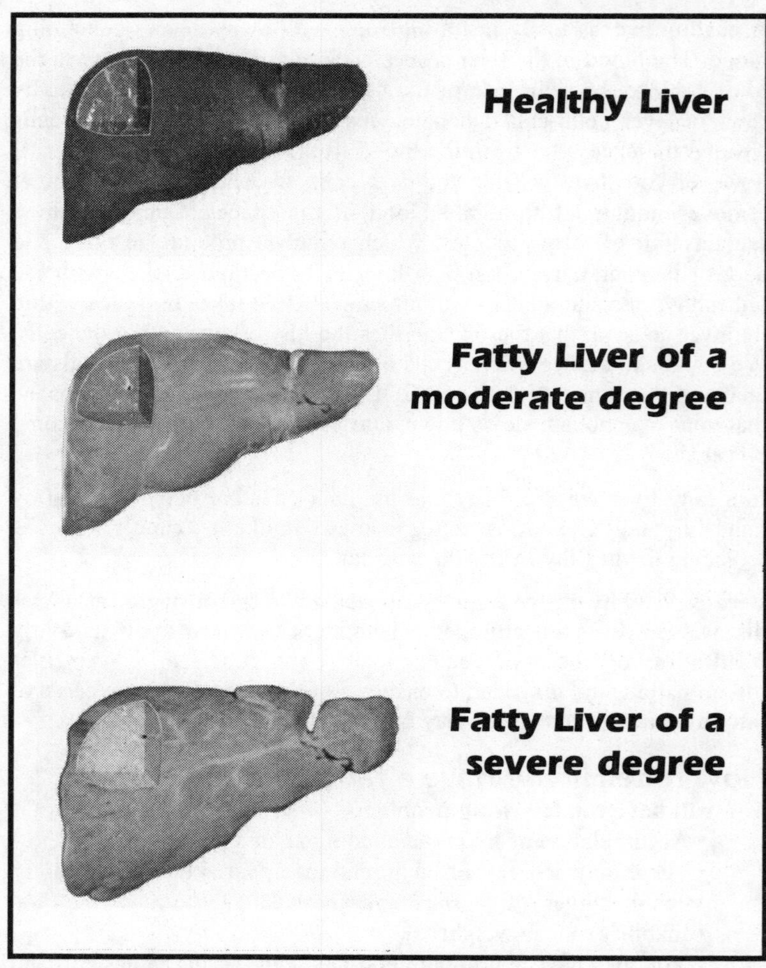

A fatty liver can be a "toxic liver"

Many environmental toxins and hormones are fat-soluble, and do not dissolve in watery fluids such as blood, bile and urine. These fat-soluble toxins can only be broken down by the liver cells, which contain enzymes to convert the fatty toxins into water-soluble forms. The liver cells perform this detoxification of fatty toxins via the phase one and two detoxification biochemical pathways - *see diagram page 65*

It is only possible for these fatty toxins to be eliminated from the body if they are converted to water-soluble waste products. Once they are water-soluble, these toxins can be eliminated from the body in watery fluids such as the bile, sweat, saliva and urine. If the liver is not able to perform its detoxification of these fatty toxins efficiently, these toxins will be deposited into the fatty areas of the body. If you have a fatty liver, large amounts of these toxins can be deposited inside the fatty liver cells where they stagnate, and further compromise the metabolic processes of the liver cells. The fatty toxins will also be drawn to other fatty areas of your body such as the brain, the hormonal glands, and fat deposits in the buttocks, abdomen, thighs, and indeed wherever you store fat. These toxins can poison the inner metabolic processes of the fat cells so that your fat cells become sluggish and inactive. It is much harder to break down these poisoned fat cells and indeed they often become cellulite.

This is why detoxification of the body can help with weight loss, as it helps to remove the toxins from the fat cells and liver cells. Once the toxins are removed the metabolic processes of the liver cells and fat cells are able to work much more efficiently, and normal fat metabolism is able to resume.

A fatty or toxic liver will cause problems with blood sugar control, as its function is impaired to some degree by the build up of fat and toxins within the liver cells. . Even slight impairment of liver function may result in a reduced ability of the liver to manufacture Glucose Tolerance factor (GTF), and insulin resistance will be aggravated by this. This leads to Syndrome X.

A fatty or toxic liver does not store glycogen as well as it should. Thus when your liver is called upon to release glucose into the blood stream from its glycogen stores, there is not enough to go around. Blood sugar levels then plummet and you start craving sugar again. This is also part of Syndrome X.

What causes fatty liver?

Fatty liver generally takes several years, and sometimes many years to develop. It is more common in overweight persons over the age of 40, but is not rare in much younger people.

The most common cause of fatty liver used to be alcohol excess, and it is still a common cause today. However, it has been overtaken by incorrect diet, as the major cause of fatty liver. The regular consumption of high amounts of refined sugar, processed snack foods, hydrogenated vegetable oils, along with greasy foods such as deep fried foods, has caused fatty liver syndrome to become very common. Many of the processed low fat foods that are consumed contain high amounts of carbohydrates in the form of added sugar, and the "plastic fats" called hydrogenated vegetable oils. The liver will convert this sugar into fat, which will be stored in the liver. It is not easy for the liver to metabolise the hydrogenated transfatty acids, as they are the wrong shape and do not fit the cell membranes properly. Thus these transfatty acids tend to accumulate in the liver. If you have a fatty liver it is important to read the nutrition panel on food labels, and to avoid foods with labels showing high amounts of hydrogenated vegetable oils and added sugar.

A lack of raw foods and vegetables and a deficiency of essential fatty acids (the good fats), can also cause fatty liver.

Raw foods and their juices contain living enzymes and nutrients that help the liver to break down fat. These foods have a cleansing effect upon the liver filter and also help the liver cells to break down and eliminate toxins. That is one of the reasons why eating raw salads and fruits, and drinking raw vegetable juices, helps with weight loss.

Essential fatty acids *(see page 150)* are vitally important for the fat burning function of the liver. The liver cell membranes and the tiny internal organs inside each liver cell are made of these essential fatty acids. The membranes and the internal organs of the liver cells have much to do with the metabolism of fats, and if they are of poor quality, your ability to regulate fat metabolism will be poor. You will not have healthy cell membranes if you lack essential fatty acids in your diet. Those who eat lots of trans-fatty acids will have problems with their cell membranes and cellular organs, as these transfatty acids do not fit into the cell membrane correctly, so you will have holes and defects in your cell membranes. This will cause the inner metabolic processes of the cells to slow down, which results in weight gain.

It is also thought that the regular consumption of artificial sweeteners, such as aspartame, will increase the risk of fatty liver. Aspartame is toxic to the liver where it is broken down into methanol (wood alcohol) and formaldehyde. Chemical artificial sweeteners may cause instability of the blood sugar levels, which will lead to hypoglycaemia and thus make you crave carbohydrates even more. If you want to have a weight problem I suggest that you use artificial chemical sweeteners on a regular basis. To help you lose weight I recommend that you avoid artificial sweeteners – *see page 134*

If the liver is repeatedly exposed to toxins such as pesticides, insecticides, organic solvents etc, and some prescription medications, liver damage may occur, which results in fatty changes in the liver.

Minimise your exposure to such toxins and keep your home environment friendly. The drugs that are most likely to cause liver damage are long term antibiotics, non-steroidal anti-inflammatory drugs, some anti-fungal drugs, and painkillers. If you have to take any of these drugs on a long-term basis please ask your doctor to check your liver function regularly with a simple blood test. You will be able to avoid liver damage and fatty liver this way. Before committing to the long-term ingestion of any drugs, ask your doctor to see the full side effect profile of the drug – you may get a shock! I have seen many people develop mysterious liver disease in adulthood, and the only antecedent factor that I could find was overexposure to drugs, especially during childhood, where the over use of antibiotics used to be wide spread.

The Cleansing Function of the Liver

The liver is the cleanser and filter of the blood stream and is of vital importance.

The liver filter can remove a wide range of microorganisms such as bacteria, fungi, viruses and parasites from the blood stream.

Infections with parasites often come from the contaminated water supplies found in large cities, and indeed other dangerous organisms may find their way into your gut and blood stream from these sources. This can cause chronic infections and poor health, so it is important to protect your liver from overload with these microorganisms. The safest thing to do is boil your water for at least 5 minutes, or drink only bottled water that has been filtered and sterilised. High loads of unhealthy microorganisms can also come from eating foods that are prepared in conditions of poor hygiene by persons who are carrying bacteria, viruses or parasites on their skin. Foods, especially meats that are not fresh or are preserved, also contain a higher bacterial load, which will overwork the liver filter if they are eaten regularly.

It is only the liver that can purify the blood stream and we only have one liver.

Toxic Overload

If the phase one and two detoxification pathways in the liver become overloaded, there will be a build up of toxins in the body. Many of these toxins are fat-soluble and incorporate themselves into fatty parts of the body where they may stay for years, if not for a lifetime. The brain and the endocrine (hormonal) glands are fatty organs, and are common sites for fat-soluble toxins to accumulate. This may result in symptoms of brain dysfunction and hormonal imbalances, such as infertility, breast pain, menstrual disturbances, adrenal gland exhaustion and early menopause. Many of these chemicals (eg. pesticides, insecticides and organic solvents) are carcinogenic and have been implicated in the rising incidence of many cancers.

If the detoxification systems within the liver are overloaded, this will cause toxins, dead cells and microorganisms to build up in the blood stream. This will then increase the workload of the immune system, which will become overloaded and irritated. The immune system will then produce excessive inflammatory chemicals, and in some cases, auto-antibodies, because it is in a hyper-stimulated state. This may lead to symptoms of immune dysfunction such as allergies, inflammatory states, swollen glands, recurrent infections, chronic fatigue syndrome, fibromyalgia or autoimmune diseases. Some of the more common autoimmune diseases are systemic lupus erythematosus (SLE), sclerosing cholangitis, primary biliary cirrhosis, Hashimoto's thyroiditis, vasculitis and rheumatoid arthritis.

Immune dysfunction is common in the chemically overloaded environment we live in today, and is exacerbated by nutritional deficiencies inherent in processed and high sugar diets. Suppressive drugs are often used to treat symptoms of immune dysfunction.

Rarely does anyone think about the liver, which seems incredible to me because it is such a powerful organ and is easily improved. Indeed the simplest and most effective way to cleanse the blood stream and thus take the load off the immune system is by improving liver function.

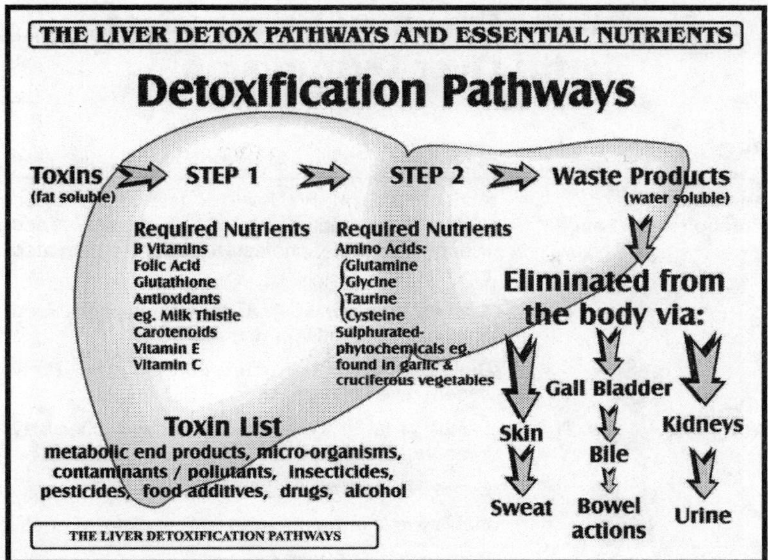

THE LIVER DETOXIFICATION PATHWAYS

Liver Dysfunction

Liver dysfunction is different to liver disease, in that the liver has not yet sustained permanent or sufficient damage to cause gross impairment of its vital functions. In those with a dysfunctional liver, the routine blood tests of liver function are often normal.

A dysfunctional liver is not working efficiently, and is overloaded, toxic or sluggish. Liver dysfunction is much more common than liver disease, and may be a forerunner to liver disease. In my experience of over 25 years of clinical medicine, I have found that approximately one in every three persons has a dysfunctional liver. Even if the level of dysfunction is only slight, it will still have a negative impact on your immune system and energy levels.

Many people suffer with the symptoms and signs of a dysfunctional liver for years, and yet the treating doctor or naturopath may not recognise the significance of these symptoms. The result is that the symptoms get treated while the underlying problem of an overloaded and toxic liver is ignored. Inevitably, the patient's symptoms deteriorate, and increasing doses of drugs such as antibiotics, anti-inflammatory medication, immune-suppressants, pain killers, and cholesterol lowering drugs etc, are needed.

Symptoms that may be associated with Liver Dysfunction

PROBLEM	SYMPTOMS
Abnormal Metabolism of Fats	• Abnormalities in the level of fats in the blood stream, for example, elevated LDL cholesterol and reduced HDL cholesterol, and elevated triglycerides.
	• Arteries blocked with fat, leading to high blood pressure, heart attacks and strokes.
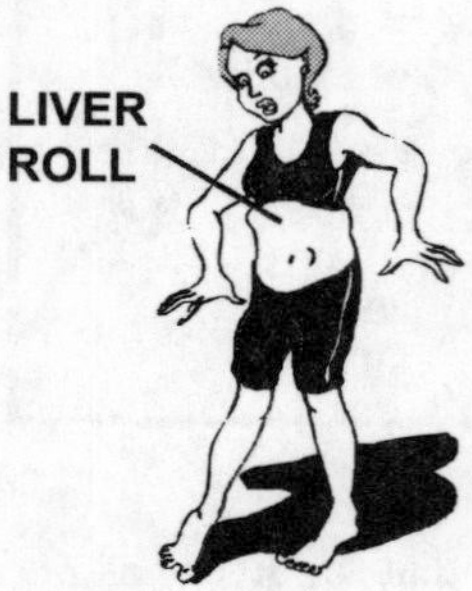	• Build up of fat in other body organs (fatty degeneration of organs).
	• Lumps of fat in the skin (lipomas and other fatty tumours).
	• Excessive weight gain, which may lead to obesity.
	• Inability to lose weight even while dieting.
	• Protuberant abdomen (pot belly).
	• Cellulite.
	• Fatty liver.
	• Roll of fat around the upper abdomen (Liver Roll)
Gastrointestinal Problems	• Indigestion and/or reflux
	• Haemorrhoids.
	• Gall stones and gall bladder disease.
	• Intolerance to fatty foods and/or alcohol
	• Nausea and vomiting attacks.
	• Abdominal bloating and flatulence (gas)
	• Irritable bowel syndrome and/or constipation
	• Discomfort over the liver - (upper right corner of abdomen & lower right rib cage).
Blood Sugar Problems	• Craving for sugar.
	• Hypoglycaemia and unstable blood sugar levels.
	• Syndrome X and type 2 diabetes is common in those with a fatty liver.

PROBLEM	SYMPTOMS
Nervous System	• Depression. • Mood changes such as anger and irritability. Metaphysically the liver is known as the "seat of anger". • Poor concentration and "foggy brain". • Overheating of the body, especially the face and torso. • Recurrent headaches (including migraine) associated with nausea.
Immune Dysfunction	• Allergies - sinus, hay fever, asthma, dermatitis, hives, etc. • Multiple food and chemical sensitivities. • Increased risk of autoimmune diseases. • Chronic Fatigue Syndrome and/or fibromyalgia • Increase in recurrent viral, bacterial and parasitic infections.
External Signs	• Coated tongue and/or bad breath • Skin rashes and/or itchy skin (pruritus). • Excessive sweating and/or offensive body odour. • Dark circles under the eyes, yellow discolouration of the eyes, and/or red swollen itchy eyes (allergic eyes). • Acne rosacea - (red pimples around the nose, cheeks and chin). • Brownish spots and blemishes on the skin (liver spots). • Red palms and soles, which may also be itchy and inflamed. • Flushed facial appearance, or excessive facial blood vessels (capillaries/veins).

NOTE: All of the above symptoms are common manifestations of a dysfunctional liver. However, they can also be due to other causes, of a more sinister nature, so, in all cases of persistent symptoms, it is vital to see your doctor.

Life saving strategies to improve your liver function

- Think of yourself as "bugs' bunny"! This means that you need to start **eating raw foods more regularly**, especially salad vegetables. All varieties of vegetables may be used in salads even avocado! Leafy greens, carrots, cucumber, shallots, onion, capsicum, coriander, parsley and indeed any vegetable may be used *– see our delicious salad recipes page 260*
  You should ideally eat raw foods with EVERY MEAL. It is quite OK to combine raw foods with cooked foods. Raw foods will improve the digestion of the meal as they contain living enzymes and antibiotics.
  Raw fruits are excellent too, but if you have Syndrome X do not overdose on huge amounts of fruits as they contain simple sugars such as fructose, which will elevate insulin levels if eaten in excessive amounts. It is generally beneficial to eat up to 4 to 5 pieces of raw fruit daily, unless you are diabetic when you will need to eat less. If you are trying to lose weight you may want to limit your pieces of fruit to no more than 2 daily until you have reached your desired weight.
  Many of my patients have told me that they only began to lose weight after they started to eat raw salads and drink raw vegetable juices. They did not change their diet in any other way and were surprised to find that raw foods made all the difference. Raw foods seem to stimulate the fat burning process especially in the liver, probably because of their cleansing effect upon the liver and lymphatic system. They also contain living enzymes and phyto-nutrients that repair damaged liver cells and help the bile to flow more freely. As bile is an important route for pumping excess fat out of the body, it is not surprising to know that raw foods and juices are so instrumental in helping us to kick start our fat loss program.

- Eat foods containing plenty of **natural organic sulphur**, and sulphur bearing amino acids. Suitable foods are eggs, cruciferous vegetables (cabbage, Brussels sprouts, cauliflower, broccoli), and vegetables from the onion family, such as onions, leeks, shallots and garlic. Sulphur helps the phase two detoxification pathways of the liver to work more efficiently, and will help weight loss and the immune system. An excellent supplemental source of organic sulphur to help the liver can be obtained by taking MSM, which stands for Methyl Sulphonyl

Methane. MSM works better when combined with vitamin C. I recommend that you take half a teaspoon twice daily mixed in raw juices.

- Start to **juice regularly**

Juices made freshly from raw vegetables have unique healing and rejuvenating properties.

I have seen raw juices work miracles in people with the following problems –

Fatty liver
Liver diseases
Obesity
Syndrome X
Inflammatory bowel disease
Chronic fatigue syndrome
Immune dysfunction
Skin problems
Recurrent infections
Arthritis

For those who feel they need an extra energy boost there is nothing better than having a raw juice everyday. It will brighten up the day by providing extra energy and endurance. Juices are unique because they allow the gut to receive very concentrated amounts of healing and powerful phyto-nutrients that could not be obtained by eating a normal amount of raw vegetables and fruits.

Raw Juices are high in -

Vitamin C, bioflavonoids, carotenoids, living plant enzymes to aid digestion, and vitamin K in green leafy vegetables. They also contain their own natural antibiotics, which make them life saving for those trying to overcome chronic infections and skin problems.

If you find the juices too strong, simply dilute them with water according to your taste. Many people with Syndrome X or a weight problem will find they will need to avoid juicing fruits. Fruit juice is high in fruit sugar (fructose), which may raise the blood sugar levels. Carrot and beetroot juice also contains high amounts of sugar and should only be used in small amounts. Small amounts of apple juice can be made (say using a small apple) to flavour bitter tasting vegetable juices. If you are diabetic then it is better to avoid fruit juices and use only vegetable juices.

Juices are a great way to take your various health powders, such as selenium yeast powders, mineral powders, liver tonic powders, MSM and vitamin C powders.

Syndrome X juice

½ cup green string beans, washed and ends cut off
3 broccoli florets, washed and sliced in half
4 Brussels sprouts – washed and base cut off
Pass all through the juicer and drink immediately

This combination can be effective in lowering blood sugar levels and improving liver function. This juice recipe will be helpful for weight loss if you have Syndrome X. If you really cannot cope with the somewhat bitter taste, add a small red apple to the juicer.

Natural Antibiotic Juice

One carrot
One cup cut cabbage
One clove garlic (may reduce amount if it is too strong)
One red radish
¼ inch fresh ginger root
½ small red apple

Pass all the above through the juicer. Take with ¼ tsp of MSM and Vitamin C powder, and this will provide an excellent natural antibiotic that may be able to get you off long-term antibiotic drugs. Olive leaf extract capsules also have natural antibiotic properties to help fight chronic infections. For more information and recipes on juicing, see my book titled "Raw Juicing can save your Life."

Syndrome X and the liver

The liver function has much to do with the development of Syndrome X

One thing that amazed me as I was doing research for Syndrome X was that none of the other researchers or experts gave much attention to the liver. Indeed as always the liver seems to be the forgotten organ and is never given the strategic importance it deserves.

The liver plays a huge and vitally important role in the regulation of carbohydrate metabolism and blood sugar control.

- It manufactures a substance called glucose tolerance factor (GTF), which helps insulin to work much more efficiently in controlling blood sugar levels. GTF facilitates the insulin-mediated transfer of glucose from the blood into the cells, and thus reduces insulin resistance.

- It stores glycogen and contains approximately 80 grams of glycogen. When blood sugar levels drop, such as in between meals, the liver breaks down the glycogen into glucose and releases the glucose into the blood stream. This prevents the blood sugar level from dropping too low and maintains a stable level of blood glucose. If this liver function is impaired, blood glucose levels can drop too low, which causes strong cravings for sugary foods. Many people with Syndrome X experience extremely strong cravings for carbohydrates.
- It manufactures glucose by a process called gluconeogenesis. The raw materials that the liver uses to synthesise glucose are lactate, pyruvate, amino acids (mainly alanine and glutamine), and glycerol from the breakdown of fat stores.

The liver plays a vitally important role in fat metabolism, which is important in the development of Syndrome X and obesity.

To put it simply one could say that the liver is the major fat burning organ in the body. It manufactures fats, recycles fats, and pumps excessive fats out of the body through the bile in to the intestines.

Fats are insoluble in watery fluids and thus are insoluble in the blood stream. In order to transport fats around the body in the blood circulation, the fats must be coated with protein. These complexes of fat and protein are called lipoproteins. The word lipid means fat.

The liver manufactures various lipoproteins, such as very low-density lipoproteins (VLDLs) and high-density lipoproteins (HDLs). VLDLs are bad news for your blood vessels, whereas the HDLs have a protective effect on your blood vessels. The HDLs go out into the circulation and scavenge the bad cholesterol, and then bring it back to the liver where it is recycled into other fats, or pumped out of the body through the bile.

The fat called triglyceride is manufactured in the liver and is incorporated into VLDLs.

Pure cholesterol is mainly manufactured in the liver and is a fat vital to healthy body function. Cholesterol is the raw material for the body's production of natural steroid and sex hormones, and is required to form cell membranes and the myelin sheath around the nerves.

Many people have been brain washed into thinking that any dietary cholesterol is unhealthy, bad, dangerous and to be avoided at all costs.

Food labels that proudly state that “this is a low fat food” or that “this is a cholesterol free food” reinforce this fallacy. This is no big deal, as if you do not eat any cholesterol, your liver will manufacture all the cholesterol that you need. If you have a healthy liver, the balance of the good cholesterol (HDL) and the bad cholesterol (LDL) and the triglycerides will be favourable in the vast majority of cases. It is not so much the avoidance of dietary cholesterol that is important, but the state of your liver that is important, when it comes to keeping your blood fats in a healthy balance and avoiding Syndrome X.

Liver Tonics

If you have a sluggish metabolism and/or a fatty liver a good liver tonic in powder or capsule form can improve your liver function. These liver tonics support the function of the liver and help to improve its detoxification and fat burning functions.

The liver is the most strategic organ in the body and therefore everyone, even the fit and healthy, need to take care of their liver in this chemical day and age.

A good liver tonic should contain the following ingredients:

• St. Mary's Thistle (Milk Thistle)

St. Mary’s Thistle, also known as Silybum Marianum, is a herb with remarkable liver protective effects. Research has shown that Milk Thistle can protect against some severe liver toxins. Many studies have been done in humans, which prove the healing and protective effects of this herb. Silymarin functions as an antioxidant and reduces damage to liver cell membranes. Silymarin can increase the quantity of the powerful liver protector called glutathione, and improves protein synthesis in the liver. *(REF. 15)*

• Taurine

Taurine is a sulphur bearing amino acid that should be present in all liver tonics. Taurine is essential for the healthy production of bile, and the liver uses it to conjugate toxins and drugs to excrete them from the body through the bile. It helps the liver to excrete excessive cholesterol out of the body through the bile, and thus is an aid for weight control and the prevention of atherosclerosis. Taurine is made from the amino acids methionine and cysteine, and is called the detoxifying amino acid. It is one of the most abundant sulphur-based amino acids in the body. It is an essential component of cell membranes, where it plays a role in stabilising transport across cell membranes and provides anti-oxidant protection. *(REF. 16)*

• Psyllium

Psyllium is an excellent source of soluble mucilloid fibre, and has been shown to lower cholesterol levels by 14 to 20% after 8 weeks. The largest trial conducted looking at the benefits of psyllium fibre was carried out at the University of Newcastle, Australia, and found that psyllium is probably the best cholesterol lowering fibre available.

• Dandelion

Dandelion known as Taraxacum Officinale, has been used by diverse cultures for centuries to help those with liver and biliary complaints. It is able to stimulate digestion and the production and flow of bile. This is because it contains bitter substances such as taraxacin and inulin.

Dandelion has laxative and diuretic actions and also stimulates the flow of bile. It is useful for liver and gall bladder inflammation and congestion, as well as jaundiced states. The Australian Journal of Medical Herbalism, Vol 3 (4), 1991 refers to two studies which demonstrate the liver healing properties of dandelion. They found that dandelion successfully treats hepatitis, liver swelling, and indigestion in those with inadequate bile secretion.

• Globe Artichoke

Globe Artichoke also known as Cynara scolymus is a bitter tonic with liver-protective and liver-restorative actions. Clinical studies have established its value in lowering blood cholesterol and nitrogen waste products of metabolism. *(REF. 17)*

Globe Artichoke is of use as a liver restorative in cases of liver insufficiency and damage, poor digestion, gallstones, and chronic constipation.

• Other Ingredients

Slippery Elm Bark powder produces a soothing effect upon the mucous membranes of the gastrointestinal tract. It produces temporary relief from excess gastric acidity and reflux.

Carrot, Beetroot, Alfalfa and Barley leaf are added to provide a boost of chlorophyll, antioxidants, carotenoids and fibre.

Lecithin helps the liver to metabolise fats and reduces high cholesterol levels. It contains phosphatidylcholine, which is beneficial for the cell membranes in the liver.

Peppermint is a carminative and is said to relax the oesophageal sphincter and intestinal muscles. It is useful in cases of travel and morning sickness, irritable bowel syndrome and as a digestive aid.

Liver tonics containing the above ingredients are helpful for the following -

- As a comprehensive general liver tonic
- An aid for weight reduction and fat burning
- An aid for those with high cholesterol and/or triglycerides
- Gall bladder dysfunction and gall stones
- Fluid retention and abdominal bloating
- Constipation (the powder is more effective than the capsules as a laxative)
- Irritable Bowel Syndrome
- Relief of digestive disorders
- Bad breath and coated tongue
- To rid the body of waste and promote elimination via a cleansing effect on the bowel

Directions for use:
It is recommended to take the Liver tonic powder in the initial stages for a 4-week period and then continue with the capsules. The reason for starting with the powder is because it contains more fibre to assist in the early stages of liver and bowel cleansing.

Standard doses are one teaspoon of the powder twice daily in fresh juices, or two capsules twice daily with food.

Commence with half this dose for the first two weeks, then begin the full dose. While taking the powder or capsules ensure that you increase the intake of pure water to 8 to 12 glasses daily. This water should be drunk gradually throughout the day. Raw vegetable juices are also vitally important for liver health. This increased fluid intake will assist the detoxification and weight loss process.

Stronger Liver tonics

Powerful synergistic formulas are available that have been designed to support the metabolic detoxification pathways within the liver. They contain specific ingredients that can stimulate the repair and renewal of damaged liver cells. They also enhance the liver's ability to break down toxic chemicals via the Phase One and Phase Two detoxification pathways.

A powerful liver tonic should contain the following -

- **St. Mary's Thistle (Milk Thistle)** *see page - 72*

- **Glutamine**

The amino acid glutamine is required for phase 2 detoxification in the liver. Glutamine is converted in the body into glutamic acid, which along with the amino acids cysteine and glycine, is converted into the powerful liver protector glutathione. Glutathione is essential for liver phase two conjugation reactions used during the detoxification of drugs and toxic chemicals. *(REF. 32)*

- **Glycine**

This amino acid performs more biochemical functions than any other amino acid. It is required for the synthesis of bile salts and is used by the liver to detoxify chemicals in the phase 2 detoxification pathways.

- **Taurine** *see page - 72*

- **Cysteine**

Cysteine is a sulfur bearing amino acid and is essential for the phase 2-detoxification pathway in the liver. It is a precursor of glutathione, which is needed to break down pollutants and toxins and has powerful antioxidant effects. Aldehydes, which are toxic breakdown products of alcohol, and rancid fats, are partially neutralised by cysteine.

- **Antioxidants**

The most important liver antioxidants are, vitamin E, vitamin C, and natural carotenoids. Green tea also has useful antioxidant properties. These help to prevent free radicals from oxidising the cell membranes in the liver, which prevents cell damage. During the detoxification of drugs and chemicals, a large amount of free radicals are generated in the liver, and antioxidants are needed to prevent these from causing liver damage. *(REF. 18)*

- **B-group Vitamins and their associated factors**

The B-group Vitamins - B 1, B 2, B 3, B 5, B 6, B 12, Folic Acid, Biotin, and Inositol should be present in a powerful liver tonic.

These vitamins are essential for energy metabolism in the liver as well as the liver's detoxification pathways. Vitamin B 12 is required for the liver to perform methylation, which inactivates the hormone oestrogen, and enhances the flow of bile.
Interestingly many strict vegans are deficient in Vitamin B 12 and Taurine, which can result in liver dysfunction.

- **Lecithin**

Lecithin contains healthy fats, which are required for the functional and structural integrity of cell membranes. Lecithin is composed of choline, linoleic acid and inositol. A choline deficiency promotes liver damage, which can be corrected with lecithin supplements. Choline is helpful for those with fatty liver and high cholesterol.

- **Zinc**

This mineral is part of the powerful antioxidant enzyme called Superoxide Dismutase (SOD). Zinc is vital for the efficient functioning of the cellular immune system needed to fight infections from viruses, parasites, and fungal microorganisms.

- **Broccoli powder**

Broccoli is a cruciferous vegetable, which contains healing phyto-nutrients such as indoles, thiols, and sulphur compounds, which enhance the detoxification pathways.

You may take all these ingredients individually or combined together, which makes it much easier to take and much more affordable.

For more information on the liver call the Health Advisory Line on free call 1800 151052.

Powerful Liver tonics are helpful for —

- Fatty liver induced by alcohol, diabetes or poor diet.
- Increased protection for people who work in high risk occupations such as painters, hairdressers, motor mechanics, agricultural workers, foundry workers, plumbers, plant and transport operators and some process and factory workers, who are exposed to high loads of potential liver toxins such as petrochemicals insecticides and solvents. Ensure that you use safe work practises to protect your liver, if you are working around potential liver toxins.
- Unstable blood sugar levels and hypoglycaemia, causing strong sugar cravings leading to poor dietary choices.
- Support for those people who are poor detoxifiers of drugs, or have multiple chemical or food allergies.
- Syndrome X
- An aid for weight reduction and fat burning
- An aid for those with high cholesterol and/or triglyceride levels
- Gall bladder dysfunction and gall stones
- Digestive problems & irritable bowel syndrome

Adverse reactions:

If the patient is very toxic the initial use of the full dose of a powerful liver tonic may cause excessive release of toxins resulting in headaches, nausea or diarrhoea. Thus it is important to begin with a lower dose to avoid these unpleasant reactions. It is important to drink at least 10 glasses of pure water during the day.

5

CHAPTER Five

Protect your children from obesity

Protect your children from obesity

Childhood obesity is rising to epidemic proportions and is alarming health care professionals and parents. Around one in four or five children are overweight or obese, and many do not exercise. Recently a study in the UK found that 25% of children do no exercise at all, and this is a similar scenario in Australia. In the USA over the past 40 years, obesity has increased 54% among children aged 6 to 11, and 40% among adolescents. According to a study by the University of North Carolina, obese children are 53 times more likely to have Syndrome X, which often precedes type 2 diabetes. This could put many children on the fast track for developing type 2 diabetes by adolescence or early adulthood.

Our children will be at an increased risk of developing cardiovascular disease and diabetes because of their increasing weight, if we do not change this worrying trend.

It is much harder for children today, as the presence of fast food has become ubiquitous. In many places you cannot walk more than 15 metres without being exposed to easily accessible food. There is enticing fast food at the petrol station, the shopping centres and the video stores.

You may be surprised that I not infrequently receive pleas for help from mothers whose young children have a fatty liver. Thirty years ago it was extremely rare to find fatty livers in children, as this condition was usually seen in older persons who had a long history of alcohol abuse or obesity.

Indeed not long ago I received a phone call from one of my naturopaths, regarding a mother who was highly distressed about her 9-year-old son who had a severe case of fatty liver. It was so severe that she had been told her son would require a liver transplant. It is incredible to think that such a young boy would be suffering with a fatty liver. When I spoke to this woman I asked her about the child's diet. She told me that her son hated eating anything raw, and would not eat any fruits or vegetables at all. His diet mainly consisted of bread and margarine, chips, sweet cereals, hamburgers and snack foods high in sugar and hydrogenated vegetable oils. He would eat a little meat, but preferred fatty hamburger meat and mincemeat, and would not drink water. He only drank soft fizzy drinks, so she had started to give him diet drinks full of aspartame. The boy was considerably overweight and carried most of the weight in the abdominal area. It is hard for children like this who have been brought up on sugar and artificial fats, as their taste buds have become distorted.

Another case history of interest involves a mother in the USA, who E-mailed me for help with her six year old daughter who was 48 inches (1.2 metres) tall and weighed 85 pounds (40 kilograms). This child carried her excess weight in the trunk and abdomen, and was found to have elevated liver enzymes during a screening test for urinary incontinence. She was tested for all sorts of liver disease and was eventually found to have a fatty liver on an ultrasound scan. This very young child was found to have the chemical imbalances of Syndrome X – namely elevated triglycerides and insulin levels, although thankfully her blood sugar levels were still within normal limits. She did suffer with the adult problem of heartburn due to reflux of stomach acids caused by her enlarged fatty liver pressing upon her stomach.

According to her mother, her daughter's favourite foods were ice cream, cheese, salty chips and crackers.

The child's diet was analysed by a dietician, and was found to be too high in carbohydrates (75% of her daily calories) and too low in protein.

Very recently this mother started her daughter on the Liver Cleansing Diet, as her specialist approved this diet as very helpful for her child's condition.

Children should not be placed on a calorie-restricted diet unless supervised by a dietician or doctor.

Helpful things that you can do to help your child include –

- Provide your child with a structured meal and snack plan
- Help your child to recognise true hunger and satiation
- Make healthy foods taste good and look appealing
- Make meal times at home a fun family event
- Make visits to the fast food outlets a special treat, and not a regular event
- Encourage exercise and outdoor activities
- Limit the time spent with TV and computers
- Keep fast foods and foods high in refined sugars and processed fats out of your pantry.
- Remember that the natural herbal-no-calorie-sweetener stevia can be used to partially or fully substitute for added sugar in homemade desserts. One big advantage of stevia is that it does not cause tooth decay.

6

Chapter Six

Diabetes and Syndrome X

Diabetes and Syndrome X

Research over the last decade has clearly shown a relationship between Syndrome X and the development of type 2 diabetes. The chemical imbalance of Syndrome X will often gradually worsen so that the blood sugar levels continue to rise to diabetic levels.

The chemical imbalance of Syndrome X begins with insulin resistance, meaning the body cells gradually become unresponsive to the hormone insulin.

The pancreas responds to this increasing resistance to insulin by producing extra amounts of insulin so that insulin levels rise. High levels of insulin are known as hyperinsulinaemia. This is the second stage of Syndrome X.

Eventually the pancreas is unable to compensate for the insulin resistance, and blood sugar levels rise, resulting in glucose intolerance.

The increased insulin levels help to compensate for the high blood sugar levels, however there is a price to pay for this. This is because the high insulin levels bring with them an increased risk of obesity, high blood pressure and heart disease.

Eventually the pancreas is unable to keep up with the high demand for insulin and the pancreas becomes "burnt out". Insulin levels then become inadequate in controlling the blood sugar levels and diabetes type 2 becomes apparent. Approximately one in four people with Syndrome X will go on to develop type 2 diabetes.

Diabetes

The emerging epidemic

which could break the health budget by 2005

One million Australians now have diabetes and its incidence has tripled in the last 20 years. These statistics come from a report called "The Australian Diabetes, Obesity and Lifestyle Study," which was sent to the Federal Government warning that the total cost to the nation will approximate $2 billion per annum by 2005.

The report found that the diagnoses of diabetes has surged 300 percent since 1981, when there were only 300,000 Australians aged over 25 years with type 2 diabetes. In 2001 there were 940,000 Australians with type 2 diabetes, and 60,000 with type 1 diabetes. This report was one of the first accurate national studies of diabetes prevalence, and acts as a warning to other developed countries.

The report indicates a diabetes prevalence of 7.5% of the Australian population aged 25 years and over. Even more worrying is the fact that for every diagnosed diabetic there is an undiagnosed case. Thus there are many people walking around who feel unwell because of undiagnosed diabetes and yet they have no idea that they have a serious metabolic problem.

The word diabetes means excessive urination. Before laboratory testing became available, doctors obliged to taste their patient's urine distinguished the sweet flavour of diabetes mellitus from other causes of excessive urination.

There are two different types of diabetes, which have very different characteristics. These are called type 1 and type 2 diabetes. Type 1 and type 2 diabetes are very different diseases – type 1 resulting from insulin lack, and type 2 coming from insulin resistance.

Type 1 Diabetes

Type 1 diabetes accounts for only 10% of all diabetes, and is characterised by a deficiency of the hormone insulin caused by failure of the pancreas gland to manufacture insulin. This typically occurs in young people and is thus sometimes called "juvenile onset diabetes". Type 1 diabetics must take insulin replacement in the form of regular insulin injections. Type 1 diabetes is also known as "Insulin-Dependent-Diabetes Mellitus" (IDDM)

Type 2 Diabetes

In type 2 diabetics there is sufficient insulin present. Indeed in the early stages of the disease there is often excessively high levels of insulin present, however the insulin does not work well in the body. This is because the cells are resistant to the effects of insulin, so that the insulin is unable to perform its function of transferring sugar (glucose) from the blood stream into the cells. Thus the blood sugar levels remain higher than normal causing the symptoms of fatigue and poor mental performance.

Type 2 diabetes accounts for 90% of all cases of diabetes, and typically begins in middle-aged people.

Type 2 diabetes is often referred to as "mature-onset diabetes" or "Non-Insulin-Dependent-Diabetes Mellitus" (NIDDM).

The official diagnosis of diabetes is made from an elevated level of glucose in the blood after fasting for 12 hours. The fasting blood sugar level must be above 6.1 mmol/L for a diagnosis of diabetes to be made.

However, well before this fasting blood sugar level becomes permanently elevated, there have been abnormalities in the body's control of glucose and insulin levels. Some experts in diabetes have classified 5 evolutionary stages of abnormal blood sugar metabolism, which lead to diabetes type 2. Three of these stages occur before the official diagnosis of type 2 diabetes can be made. Syndrome X consists of any or all of the first three stages.

The 5 stages of abnormal blood sugar metabolism

Stage One: Insulin resistance only

Stage Two: Insulin resistance plus high levels of insulin and normal blood sugar levels

Stage Three: Insulin resistance, high levels of insulin and abnormalities in a glucose tolerance test

Stage Four: Diabetes type 2 with high insulin levels

Stage Five: Diabetes type 2 with low insulin levels

You can see that in three of the above stages (stages 2,3, and 4) there is excessive production of insulin, which will encourage weight gain in these people. If we can intervene before stage five, simply by following a strategic eating plan and using supplements to lower insulin levels, we have the greatest chance of avoiding the evolution to long term diabetes.

Insulin is the rogue hormone that we must control to reverse these four stages of chemical imbalance, and to reverse the increasing weight gain that has accompanied them.

What are the long-term complications of Diabetes?

The long-term complications of sustained high blood sugar levels are the same in both type 1 and type 2 diabetes.

People with diabetes are 3 to 4 times more likely to die of heart disease than are non-diabetics, even when blood pressure and cholesterol levels are the same.

Diabetes can cause kidney disease, which may result in kidney (renal) failure. This can result in the need for a kidney transplant.

Diabetes causes disease of the large and small blood vessels, which impairs circulation of blood to vital organs and the limbs. This may result in infections and death of tissue requiring amputation.

The high blood sugar levels in diabetics can damage the nerves resulting in gradual degeneration of the peripheral nerves (neuropathy). This causes loss of sensation and weakness of the limbs. It may also cause bladder and bowel dysfunction.

The high blood sugar levels of diabetes may cause degeneration of the proteins in the lens of the eyes resulting in cataracts. The retina of the eyes may also be damaged resulting in diabetic retinopathy, which results in blindness.

The complications of diabetes individually or collectively result in a considerably reduced life expectancy.

7

Chapter Seven

Drugs used in Diabetes and Syndrome X

Drugs used in Diabetes and Syndrome X

Drugs used to reduce blood glucose levels

There are various drugs in this category, which work on the production and/or effectiveness of insulin in the body. They can only be prescribed by your own doctor and need to be carefully controlled.

• Sulfonylurea type of drugs

There are various types (brands) of these drugs and the generic names for these drugs include-

Tolbutamide
Glibenclamide
Glipizide
Glyburide
Glimepiride
Gliclazide
Chlorpropamide
Acetohexamide
Tolazamide

They are prescribed for diabetes type 2

Actions of Sulfonylurea-type drugs
These drugs stimulate the production and release of the hormone insulin from the pancreas gland. They only work if there are some functional cells in the pancreas gland, and are not effective if the pancreas has failed completely. The different brands of these drugs vary in their potency and the duration of their effectiveness.

Cautions with the use of the Sulfonylurea type of drugs –
Infections, emotional stress, or surgery may adversely affect the effectiveness of these drugs. Occasionally these drugs may cause excessively low blood sugar levels, which is a serious problem requiring medical attention.

Do not mix these drugs with alcohol, as this may result in throbbing headaches, shortness of breath, vomiting, flushing, thirst, dizziness, chest pains, blurred vision, low blood pressure and confusion.

The Sulfonylurea drugs can cause problems in those with diseases of the liver, kidneys or endocrine (hormonal) system, and extra caution must be exercised in these situations.

These drugs do not work like insulin and are not a replacement for insulin.

Clinical studies done in the 1960s, and confirmed in 1999, found that patients taking oral sulfonylurea drugs are more likely to have fatal heart conditions, than those patients who treat their pre-diabetic condition or diabetes with diet and lifestyle changes alone, or dietary changes plus insulin medication.

Possible side effects of the oral Sulfonylurea drugs are –
Digestive upsets and poor appetite, nausea and vomiting
Fatigue
Tingling in the hands and feet
If excessive amounts are taken, low blood sugar levels may occur, which can be a serious medical emergency requiring immediate hospital attention
Skin rashes and itching
Liver inflammation and/or jaundice

• Metformin

Metformin is a Biguanide drug and is anti-hyperglycaemic, meaning that it reduces high blood glucose levels. Different brand names of Metformin are – Diabex, Glucomet, Glucophage and Diaformin

The usual dose of Metformin is 500mg twice daily with food. This dose may need to be increased gradually to a maximum dose of 3000mg daily, although older patients generally need a smaller dosage, to prevent side effects. It is not used very much in children.

Metformin is prescribed for -

Type 2 diabetes
Syndrome X
Polycystic Ovarian Syndrome, associated with the chemical imbalances of Syndrome X

Actions of Metformin-

Lowers the amount of glucose produced by the liver
Reduces the amount of glucose absorbed from food
Helps body cells to utilise glucose more efficiently
Produces a slight reduction in blood fats

Metformin cannot be used in those with the following problems -

Heart failure

Kidney disease

Liver disease

Patients taking oral anti-diabetes drugs are more likely to develop heart disease, compared to patients taking insulin, or those treated with dietary strategies alone.

Adverse reactions and side effects to Metformin –

Diarrhoea, nausea, vomiting, abdominal bloating, appetite loss and abdominal gas. These symptoms are generally short lived and are more common when the drug is first taken. It may be necessary to reduce the dose of Metformin to alleviate these side effects.

Excessively low blood sugar levels

Skin rashes

An unpleasant metallic taste in the mouth, which is usually temporary.

Low blood levels of vitamin B 12.

A rare but serious side effect of Metformin is lactic acidosis, which is fatal in 50% of cases. The symptoms of lactic acidosis can be vague and insidious in onset. They may consist of muscular pains, feeling generally unwell and fatigued, shortness of breath, and digestive upsets. If untreated this can progress to heart arrhythmia, low blood pressure and low body temperature. You should seek medical attention immediately as lactic acidosis is a medical emergency.

The risk of lactic acidosis is increased by the following –

Advancing age

Presence of heart failure

Poor kidney function

Alcohol ingestion

Using excessive doses of Metformin

Your doctor will allow for these risk factors.

• Thiazolidinedione Drugs

These are a relatively new class of drugs developed to help those with insulin resistance and type 2 diabetes.

They include the following brands –
Pioglitazone (ACTOS)
Rosiglitazone (AVANDIA)
Troglitazone (REZULIN) – now withdrawn world-wide due to liver toxicity

These drugs may be prescribed for -
Diabetes type 2
Polycystic Ovarian Syndrome, associated with the chemical imbalances of Syndrome X

Actions of Thiazolidinedione drugs -
Reduce the amount of sugar produced by the liver
Increase the amount of sugar used by the muscles, fat and liver cells
Reduce insulin resistance
They are often taken with other anti-diabetes drugs, such as Metformin or Sulfonylurea-type drugs

Cautions with the use of Thiazolidinedione drugs -
Liver disease, as these drugs may be toxic to the liver – liver function tests must be done before prescribing these drugs
Heart failure
Caution with contraception, as these drugs can trigger ovulation in women who do not ovulate

Possible side effects are –
Weakness and fatigue
Headache
Nausea and diarrhoea
Sore throat and runny nose
Back pain
Dizziness
Very rare – jaundice, hepatitis, liver failure, death
Drug interactions are common – check with your doctor

Drugs used to lower cholesterol levels

These drugs are called hypo-lipidaemic agents, and act to reduce cholesterol and/or triglyceride levels.

The most commonly prescribed drugs are the "statin drugs", and these are available under several generic brands such as –

Fluvastatin
Simvastatin
Atorvastatin
Cerivastatin
Pravastatin
Lovastatin

These drugs are very effective at lowering raised cholesterol levels, and are prescribed where dietary and lifestyle changes have failed. However those with Syndrome X will find it very hard to lower blood fat levels, unless they know the correct dietary guidelines to follow, and also improve their liver function. Many people can avoid these drugs if they follow the correct eating plan for Syndrome X. Those patients with hereditary problems of liver fat metabolism will benefit most from these drugs, but this is a minority of all people with high cholesterol levels.

According to Dr Antonio Gotto, Dean of Cornell University Medical College, New York, 50% of the entire US adult population may need to take statin medications.
He gives the following reasons –
They are supposedly very effective
They are claimed to be safe at the usual prescribed doses
They may soon be available in the US without a prescription

Precautions when taking statin drugs –
It is important to take supplements of Coenzyme Q 10, because the statin drugs lower body levels of this vital nutrient. Coenzyme Q 10 is important for heart health.

There have been many studies showing negative health effects from statin drugs. In a report published in the Journal of the American Medical Association *(REF. 20)*, statins have been shown to cause cancer in laboratory animals. The authors of this study state "lipid-lowering drug treatment, especially with the fibrates and statins, should be avoided except in patients at high short-term risk of coronary heart disease"

The following statins – Atorvastatin, Lovastatin and Pravastatin, were shown to suppress a group of immune system cells called "helper T-cells". This immuno-suppressant effect was seen in laboratory-grown cells. This is not a good effect and I am sure that patients with high cholesterol do not want to run any risk of having their immune system suppressed. *(REF. 21)*

During a conference of the American Heart Association in Orlando, Florida, on the 11th November 2000, researchers from the University of Pittsburgh discussed their findings in patients who had lowered cholesterol levels with the drug Lovastatin, and displayed problems with attention and reflex time. Those patients with the greatest reduction in cholesterol levels displayed the worst impairment of these cognitive functions. Dutch researchers found some evidence to show there was a link between depression in men and low cholesterol levels. *(REF. 22)*

The German drug company Bayer AG, during 2001, made a decision to withdraw the statin drug called Cerivastatin from the world-wide market, after it was associated with 31 deaths in the USA from severe rhabdomyolysis associated with use of cerivastatin. Around one third of the Cerivastatin deaths occurred among patients who were also taking gemfibrozil, which is a drug used to lower triglyceride levels.

In around 1 in 1,000 people who take statin drugs, the rare muscle disease called myositis can occur. Myositis can occasionally progress to rhabdomyolysis, which is a complete breakdown of muscle tissue possibly eventuating in kidney failure and death.

There is always the potential for side effects and drug interactions when large numbers of the population rely on multiple drugs to control common diseases of affluent societies such as arthritis, diabetes, high blood pressure and elevated cholesterol.

If you are taking a statin drug to control your cholesterol levels here are some worthwhile tips –

Be on the lookout for muscle weakness, pain or tenderness, or fever.

Check the colour of your urine – if it turns brown, see your doctor.

Liver function tests are routinely done in those on statin drugs. Tests to check for muscle breakdown such as creatine kinase and creatine phosphokinase should also be done if there is any muscle weakness or tenderness.

Tell your doctor if you take any other medications, including the over the counter non-prescription variety of drugs.

8

Chapter Eight

Lets talk about diets

Lets talk about diets

Why don't all high-protein diets work the same?

Many of these diets don't work because they are too high in greasy saturated and oxidised fats, and too low in the good fats.

Many of them do not give enough emphasis on improving the liver function, which means that in the long term they will not be as effective in weight control and achieving optimal health.

High protein – high fat diets (with very low carbohydrates) will help with initial weight loss because they reduce glucose and insulin levels and often put you into a state of ketosis (fat burning). However if they are followed continually as a way of life, you can run into frustrating obstacles.

This is because of the following –

- The liver and kidneys may become overworked by having to process large amounts of protein and greasy fats. Protein is broken down in the body into urea, uric acid and ammonia, which are waste products of metabolism that must be eliminated by the kidneys via the urine. Have you ever noticed that your urine gets a strong "ammonia" type of smell the day after consuming a meal with very high amounts of animal meat or poultry? This is because of the high content of ammonia, urea and creatinine waste products in the urine from eating so much protein in one hit.
- The liver has to process dietary fats, as it is the major organ of fat metabolism. Fat contains 9 calories per gram and is a calorie-dense food that needs to be handled by the liver. Many overweight persons have a fatty liver, which cannot handle a high fat diet. In a fatty liver condition the liver cells have been partly replaced with unhealthy fatty tissue, so there are less healthy liver cells left to metabolise the fats. Thus the dietary fats cannot be broken down and recycled efficiently and will tend to accumulate in the liver as fatty tissue.
  Anytime you overwork the liver there is a high chance of weight gain, as there is less metabolic energy left over in the liver for burning fat. So we do not want to overwork our liver and kidneys. If we do, we have a high chance of staying in a weight plateau for too long, in which case we will become frustrated and give up. Also overworking the liver and kidneys makes us tired and less inclined to exercise.

Weight loss is not just about rapid loss, it is about taking off the weight and keeping it off. Furthermore we are trying to improve our general health and longevity and to achieve this, healthy liver and kidney function is vital. So we do not want to be slim and unhealthy with an overworked liver. This is why balance is so important, and in my eating program you will achieve the correct balance of nutrients to stimulate fat burning. This dietary balance will also assist the production of healthy blood fats and improve your liver and kidney function. You will not be presenting the liver and kidneys with a daunting workload of having to process excessive amounts of protein and greasy fats.

Many high protein diets allow you to eat unlimited amounts of dairy products, fried meats, fatty meats, smoked meats, preserved meats (ham, bacon, pizza meats, smoked meats, sausage etc), and do not differentiate between the good proteins and bad proteins. Preserved meats are not fresh, are higher in bacteria, contain toxic preservatives and their contained fats have been oxidised by the air and processing. These types of meats will generate the production of free radicals in your body, which can damage the liver. You should only eat very fresh lean meats, and if you can find it, organic poultry is better. This is because it is free of fattening hormones.

The risk of coronary heart disease may be higher in susceptible persons who stay on a high-protein high-fat diet for too long because the consumption of saturated fat is too high.

Many high-protein high-fat diets do not differentiate between the good and the bad fats, which is risky for your liver and cardiovascular system. If you consume excessive amounts of saturated fat you run a higher risk of increasing the bad LDL-cholesterol in your blood. We know that people who have both elevated LDL-cholesterol and Syndrome X have the worst risk of heart disease.

Many high protein diets allow you to eat lots of cheese, cream, butter, fatty meats and fried meats, which are very high in saturated fat. In the long term this is unbalanced and risky and is not a healthy way of eating for life extension.

In my eating plan I allow you to eat a reasonable amount of saturated fat from specific foods, as long as it is fresh, not deep-fried and not processed.

Why don't conventional low-fat low-calorie diets work?

These diets do not work because they are too low in protein and too low in the good fats, and too high in carbohydrates.

I have seen many people become yoyo dieters on low-calorie fad diets because they are consuming too much sugar, sweet drinks, sweet low fat yoghurts, artificial sweeteners and refined carbohydrates.

Temporary weight loss may occur because the daily calories are so low, but the very low caloric intake causes the metabolic rate to slow down, so that when you come off the diet, your metabolic rate is at an all time low. So once you begin to eat normally and increase the calories, you will gain weight more rapidly then ever before. You then start to feel guilty for not having enough will power or motivation. Successful weight loss is not so much about "will power" but "know-how" – you need the right tools to avoid the chemical imbalance that causes the disturbance in your metabolism. It is not how much you eat, but what you eat that's most important! If you eat the right foods in the right combinations you do not have to deprive yourself of satisfying meals that produce a sense of fulfilment. If we minimise the high GI carbohydrates you will not have to obsessively count calories or grams of fat and yet you can still lose weight and feel satisfied.

Dietary protein and fat does not require much insulin to process, whereas refined carbohydrates do. A diet predominantly obtained from low - fat high - GI carbohydrates will increase insulin levels, and remember it is the insulin excess that makes you fat!

Low-calorie, high carbohydrate diets cause a series of chemical imbalances that make it difficult to burn stored fat.

Low-fat low-calorie diets usually cause instability of blood sugar levels, which results in fatigue and cravings for more carbohydrates. It is the fatigue and cravings that will sabotage your efforts to stay with a healthy way of eating.

I had one patient who had been trying to lose weight for 25 years on low calorie diets and was a typical yoyo dieter. She could not stay on a diet for longer then 2 weeks because of extreme tiredness and cravings, which made her become obsessed with sweet foods. She would hide these foods so she could not get at them and avoided socialising. She had come to accept chronic fatigue as a way of life, and gave up the idea of ever being slim and healthy.

I started her on my eating program and she lost her cravings and had more energy than she had experienced in years. She started to lose weight around her abdomen and lost her bloated feeling, which gave her a renewed sense of hope. A few weeks later as her confidence returned, she attended a weekend conference, and decided to enjoy the lunch of high carbohydrate foods provided. She thought that surely only one episode of eating high carbohydrate - refined foods would not cause her any problems. In the middle of the afternoon her blood sugar dropped during a lecture presentation, and she was woken up by the lady sitting next to her, as her loud snoring was making it difficult for others to hear the lecture. She was mortified and realised that her metabolism was profoundly affected by what she ate. If she had been able to eat protein foods such as fresh meats, eggs, nuts, beans and seeds along with vegetables and salad, she would have been able to enjoy the seminar and avoid acute embarrassment.

9

Chapter Nine

Carbohydrates

Carbohydrates

Carbohydrates are different forms of simple sugars linked together in polymers.

Many people do not understand what carbohydrates are. They will often say carbohydrates are confined to cakes, bread, sweets or pasta. Yes its true that these foods are high in carbohydrates, but fruits and vegetables also contain some carbohydrate. If you were to eat huge amounts of fruit and starchy vegetables every day you would be getting excessive carbohydrate, which would be absorbed as glucose and could be turned into fat. However it is difficult to eat huge amounts of unprocessed carbohydrates because they are high in fibre and take much longer to eat. Conversely, it is very easy to eat huge amounts of refined carbohydrates, as they are low in fibre and are very condensed, so that large amounts of sugar are found in much smaller portion sizes of food.

Carbohydrate generally comes from plant foods such as cereals, grains, flour, cane sugar, fruits and vegetables. Dairy products contain a carbohydrate called lactose, which is milk sugar.

• Complex carbohydrates

Complex carbohydrates are much better to eat than simple or refined carbohydrates. Complex carbohydrates do not cause a rapid rise in blood sugar levels, as they are more slowly absorbed than simple carbohydrates. They are absorbed even more slowly if they are eaten with some protein and fat. Because complex carbohydrates are starchier, they are also more filling and so satisfy the hunger for longer. Be careful when choosing complex carbohydrates, as you do not want breads and pasta made with white flour and sugar and you should choose brown or wild rice over white rice. In other words, choose the unprocessed variety of complex carbohydrates. Food made with white flour and white sugar has had all the fibre and vitamins/minerals removed from it and is of poor nutritional value.

Complex carbohydrates are generally starchy foods and are found in such things as –

Whole grains– unprocessed
Whole grain bread
Wholegrain flour products such as pasta and buckwheat noodles
Corn
Legumes – lentils, beans, peas (legumes are also a good source of protein especially when combined with nuts and seeds and grains).

Starchy vegetables such as potato, sweet potato, pumpkin, squash, turnips, parsnips, carrots, beetroots, green peas. These starchy vegetables are higher in carbohydrates than green vegetables, but are also high in fibre, vitamins, minerals, essential fatty acids and anti-oxidant phyto-nutrients, and are thus a healthy source of carbohydrates.

Green and leafy vegetables are low in carbohydrates and can be eaten freely to fill up on. They are excellent for the liver and bowel, and some of these vegetables such as green beans and Brussels sprouts can lower blood sugar and insulin levels. Fill up on generous serves of broccoli, green beans, cabbage, Brussels sprouts, spinach, salad greens, collard greens, and anything green and leafy.

• Simple carbohydrates

These are very high in pure sugars (such as glucose), and their intake needs to be controlled. Other simple sugars are fructose, maltose and lactose. If the substance ends in "ose" it's a simple sugar, which means it's a simple carbohydrate, the intake of which needs to be controlled.

Simple carbohydrates are found in –
Pure sugar (glucose)
Fructose (found in fruits)
Maltose (found in beer)
Lactose (found in cow's milk and some of its products).
Honey
Jam
Sweets and candies
Cakes
Sweet biscuits
White flour
Maple syrup
Corn syrup
Soft drinks

Fruit juices are high in sugar and are best avoided as the juicing process removes the fibre and leaves behind the sugar. Orange, apple, mango, banana, pineapple, grape and prune juice, are high in simple sugars, which are rapidly absorbed to elevate blood sugar levels. If you are making a fresh vegetable juice for yourself, you may add a small quantity of freshly expressed fruit juice to temper the flavour, but keep it to a minimum amount. Diabetics should avoid fruit juices.

Fresh fruits are the best source of refined carbohydrates, as they are high in vitamins, minerals and fibre, which reduces their rate of absorption, so they do not elevate the blood sugar levels so dramatically. Most of their calories come from simple sugars such as fructose and glucose, so you cannot eat unrestricted amounts of fruits.

Canned fruits may be very high in sugar and the fruit has lost a lot of its nutritional value.

Some dried fruit is also high in sugar and should only be eaten in small amounts. It is best substituted with fresh fruit.

What happens to carbohydrate when you eat it?

Carbohydrate is absorbed into the blood stream in the form of glucose. The brain has a high need for glucose as its primary source of energy and does not require insulin to get at this carbohydrate. The brain is a glutton for glucose, and uses more than two thirds of the circulating blood glucose while you are resting. Thus you need a continual supply of glucose to avoid brain damage and dysfunction. If there is excess glucose in the blood over and above the body's immediate energy needs, the excess glucose will be stored in the form of glycogen. Glycogen is a long chain of glucose molecules linked together.

The body has two storage sites for glycogen – the muscles and the liver cells. The liver glycogen is most accessible to be broken down into glucose to meet the requirements of the brain for immediate energy. That is why the liver function is so important in keeping blood sugar levels and brain function stable. However the liver's capacity to store glycogen is not unlimited, and can be depleted within 12 hours, if no food is eaten. The capacity of the liver to store glycogen and release it efficiently into the blood stream under times of need can be greatly reduced in those with a fatty liver or liver dysfunction, as there are not enough healthy liver cells present to store the required amount of glycogen. In such cases blood sugar levels may fluctuate erratically. If the liver is unable to store excess blood glucose in the form of glycogen, the glucose may be converted into fat, which explains why a dysfunctional liver can lead to weight excess.

What happens when you eat excess amounts of carbohydrates?

If you eat too much carbohydrate, you will exceed the glycogen storage capacity of the liver and muscle cells. In the average person there is around 300 to 400 grams of carbohydrate stored as glycogen in the muscle cells, and 60 to 90 grams in the liver. The liver's stored glycogen is equivalent to around three average sweet energy bars, and is not a lot when you think that this is all there is to keep your brain functioning normally.

Once the capacity of your muscles and liver to store glycogen is full, the remaining glucose must be converted to triglyceride fat and is stored as body fat in your adipose tissues.

So even though you are eating **fat free** carbohydrates, any excess carbohydrate must be converted into fat. Yes excess sugar is turned into fat and excessive amounts of high - carbohydrate **fat-free foods** can be terribly **fattening!**

You do not need to eat any fat to become fat!

Eating high amounts of refined carbohydrates will cause a rapid rise in blood sugar levels, which will in turn stimulate the pancreas gland to secrete high levels of insulin. Insulin will convert the excess glucose into triglyceride fat, which will be stored as body fat.

Thus insulin is a fat storing hormone!

Excess carbohydrates send a hormonal signal to the body to store fat in our fatty tissues such as the abdomen, buttocks, thighs, and also inside organs such as the liver and pancreas. Thus we may develop fatty organs with fat accumulating in the liver, pancreas, spleen, heart and skin. Yes we can become a warehouse for fat simply because the high carbohydrate intake stimulates excessive amounts of the fat storing hormone insulin. High levels of insulin also send signals to your cells not to release any stored fat. This makes it very difficult for your body to use its own stored fat for energy.

So the high levels of insulin not only make you fatter, they make sure that you stay fat!

High levels of the hormone insulin will also cause erratic fluctuations in blood sugar levels, and when blood sugar levels become low, you will crave carbohydrates. **Thus insulin stimulates hunger.**

10

Chapter Ten

Glucagon and Insulin

Glucagon and Insulin

These two hormones are produced by the pancreas gland and together regulate sugar and fat metabolism. These two hormones have a huge influence on your tendency to gain weight.

Glucagon has the opposite effect of insulin in the body. Glucagon stimulates the burning and breakdown of fatty tissues. In contrast to insulin, which promotes the storage of fat, glucagon helps the body to burn fat stores for energy.

In summary the effects of the hormone glucagon are –

It increases the burning of body fat stores for energy
It converts fat and protein to glucose
It pushes your metabolism into the fat burning zone
It raises low blood sugar levels
It decreases the production of cholesterol and triglycerides in the body
It reduces fluid retention

Action	Insulin	Glucagon
Glucose production by the liver	reduced	increased
Fat burning (lipolysis)	reduced	increased
Ketogenesis	reduced	increased

Insulin exerts exactly the opposite effect to glucagon in the body, and thus it is better for those with a weight problem to find that their scale tips in the favour of glucagon and not insulin.

Thus glucagon and insulin are the two sides of the scale and need to be in balance for healthy metabolism.

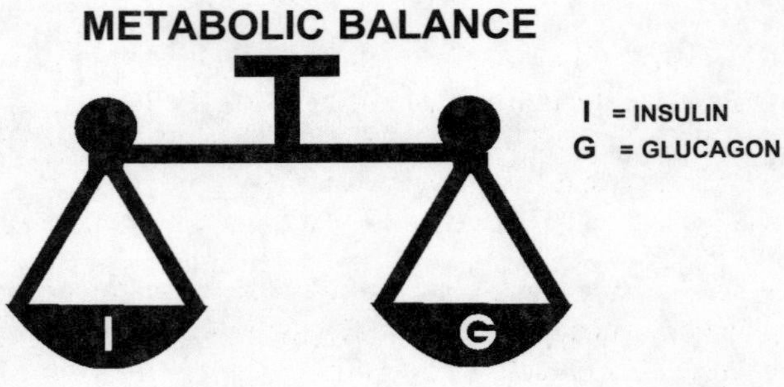

What we eat has the most pronounced effect upon our insulin and glucagon ratio.
This is summarised in the chart below -

FOOD CATEGORY	INSULIN LEVELS	GLUCAGON LEVELS
Carbohydrate	5	0
Protein	2	2
Fat	0	0
Protein & Fat	2	2
High protein & low carbohydrate	2	1
Carbohydrate & fat	4	0
High carbohydrate & low protein	9	1

From this chart you can see that dietary carbohydrate eaten by itself, has a powerful effect in raising insulin levels. This adverse effect on insulin is at its worst when meals containing large amounts of refined carbohydrates with very low protein content are consumed.

My eating plan and supplement program for Syndrome X has been designed to normalise body insulin levels, and maximise glucagon levels, so that these two crucial hormones of metabolism will remain in balance. Only then can fat burning take precedence over fat storage. Furthermore by correcting the balance of these two hormones we are treating the cause of Syndrome X. There will also be a correction in the other symptoms of Syndrome X – namely high blood pressure, high cholesterol levels and blood sugar instability. Another great benefit is that your cravings for carbohydrates will be much less, if not completely gone.

What happens when you burn body fat?

When your insulin levels are low your fat cells release free fatty acids, which are a major source of energy for your heart and skeletal muscles. Once you eat carbohydrate your glucose and insulin levels go up, and the insulin suppresses the release of fatty acids from your fat cells. Thus we can say that high levels of insulin stop you burning body fat for energy.

When you burn stored body fat it breaks down into free fatty acids and glycerol, which are then broken down into substances called ketone bodies. This process of fat burning is known as lipolysis and cannot occur without the formation of ketones.

Unless you are an insulin – dependent diabetic, there is nothing bad about forming ketones in your body, as ketones are just a sign of using body fat for fuel rather than glucose.

Ketones can be used as fuel by most parts of the body including the heart and brain. The body cannot efficiently burn ketones for energy without the presence of adequate carbohydrates. Thus on a very low carbohydrate diet it is difficult for the body to use the ketones for energy, and the excess ketones are excreted from the body in the urine, the faeces and the breath. This may give a slightly sweet smell to the breath, which is known as an “acetone breath”.

It is not dangerous to form ketones in your body unless you are an insulin-dependent diabetic. Indeed ketones are normal energy sources for many parts of the body.

The lower the dietary carbohydrate intake is, the faster will be the rate of fat burning and elimination of ketones. By liberating and excreting ketones from your body, you are eliminating the by-products of burning your unwanted fat. This is a very easy way to lose weight because you are eliminating the breakdown products of body fat, without your body having to use them for energy. Thus your body will utilise other sources of energy either from your diet, or by burning more of its fat stores, to provide the fuel it needs to keep your metabolism going. Indeed by reducing dietary carbohydrates it is possible to redirect your metabolic pathways. This is because you are not consuming enough carbohydrates to equal your energy expenditure and must therefore burn your stored body fat to supply your energy needs. A ketogenic diet is a diet where the dietary carbohydrate intake is so low that the body burns its fat stores for energy, which leads to the production of ketones in the body.

A ketogenic diet creates a new metabolic pathway for supplying the body with energy by making you a fat burner instead of a carbohydrate burner. For many people this is the most effective and easy initial way to start the weight loss process.

Ketosis

In those who are fasting or following a very low carbohydrate diet (less than 40 grams per day), the metabolic state of ketosis may occur in the body. Some people will need to consume less than 20grams of carbohydrate per day to enable ketosis to begin. In the state of ketosis your body will be burning its stored fat for energy instead of carbohydrates. You should not feel hungry, as most people do on a low-fat high-carbohydrate diet.

Ketosis is recognisable because there are measurable levels of ketones in the blood, urine, stools and the breath. It is possible to use urine test strips (Ketostix), which test for the presence of ketones in the urine. The Ketostix result gives you an indication of the amount of ketones you are excreting from your body, and thus your degree of fat burning (lipolysis). If there are ketones present in the urine, the test strips turn a pink to purple colour, depending upon the amount of ketones present. The more ketones present in the urine, the darker will be the purple colour.

Results of Ketostix

Colour	Meaning
Pink (1.5 or small)	You are burning fat gradually
Purple (4 to 16)	You are burning fat efficiently, but can eat slightly more carbohydrate if you feel tired
Trace (negative)	You are eating too many carbohydrates to be in ketosis

TABLE 3

The test strips are available under the brand name of Keto-stix designed for low carbohydrate dieters, or to warn of ketoacidosis in diabetics.

Do the urine testing twice daily. The end of the Ketostix strip is placed into a mid-steam specimen of urine, after it has been collected in a jar. If you are following an extremely low carbohydrate diet (less than 20 grams per day), you will show ketones in your urine indicating that you are burning fat and not glucose for energy. Generally speaking you will have enough carbohydrate stored as glycogen in your body for only 48 hours, and after you have used it all up, you will enter a state of ketosis.

If your urine strips do not turn pink to purple on a low carbohydrate diet, this is nothing to worry about. As long as you are losing weight and feeling well, the program in this book is still working efficiently. This means that you are still burning fat and producing ketones, but only small quantities of ketones, which are insufficient to change the colour of the test strips.

Warning

If you decide to go on a very low carbohydrate diet (less than 40 grams of carbohydrate per day), you **MUST** do this under the supervision of your own doctor and/or naturopath. This applies to everyone and especially to those who are obese (with a body mass index of over 30), those with medical problems such as heart disease, kidney disease, or any other chronic medical problem. You will need to drink at least 2.5 litres of water daily while in the state of ketosis.

When first entering the state of ketosis you may experience unpleasant symptoms due to detoxification. These may include headaches, nausea, fatigue or dizziness. In those with a tendency to gout, a ketogenic diet may increase the risk of an acute attack of gouty arthritis. This is because the blood uric acid levels increase, as the uric acid competes with ketones for excretion in the urine. High uric acid levels increase the risk of kidney problems, so those with impaired kidney function should not follow a ketogenic diet unless it is recommended and supervised by their own doctor.

Drinking plenty of water and taking a liver tonic powder may reduce the detoxification symptoms of a ketogenic diet.

Diabetics (especially insulin dependent diabetics) are not able to follow a ketogenic diet (extremely low carbohydrate diet) unless their own doctor advises it. This is because it can destabilise their blood sugar control and lead to dangerous metabolic problems.

11

Chapter Eleven

Glycaemic Index of Foods

Glycaemic Index of Foods

The Glycaemic Index (GI) measures the effect of a specific food upon your blood sugar levels after you eat it.

The standard against which all foods are measured on the Glycaemic Index (GI) scale is pure glucose, which is given a GI rating of 100. Every other food is measured on a scale from 0 to 100 depending upon its effect on blood sugar levels.

Different types of carbohydrate foods will have very different effects upon your blood sugar levels and therefore your insulin levels. Carbohydrates cause blood sugar and insulin levels to rise more rapidly than any other types of foods. This applies especially to refined carbohydrates, which are rapidly absorbed from the gut into the blood stream. However if a carbohydrate food is absorbed slowly from the gut, less insulin is required. It is not just the ***amount*** of carbohydrate you eat that's important, it's the ***type*** of carbohydrate you eat that also determines the magnitude of the rise in blood sugar levels.

How do we determine the Glycaemic Index (GI) of a specific food?

- A person is given an amount of the test food (lets say its spaghetti this time that we are testing), which equals 50 grams of pure carbohydrate. In the case of spaghetti the test person would have to eat 200grams of spaghetti in order to supply 50 grams pure carbohydrate. 50 grams of pure carbohydrate is found in 3 tablespoons of pure sugar(glucose) powder.
- During the 2 hours after the test food is eaten, a sample of blood is taken every 15 minutes during the first hour, and then every 30 minutes during the second hour.
- The blood sugar levels are measured from these blood samples.
- The blood sugar level is plotted on a graph and the area under the curve is calculated using a special formula - *see diagram 3- page 117.*
- The person's response to the test food (spaghetti on this occasion) is compared with his/her blood sugar response after eating 50grams of pure sugar (glucose), which is used as the reference standard.

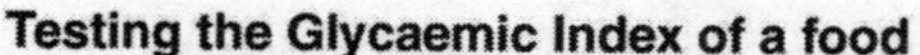

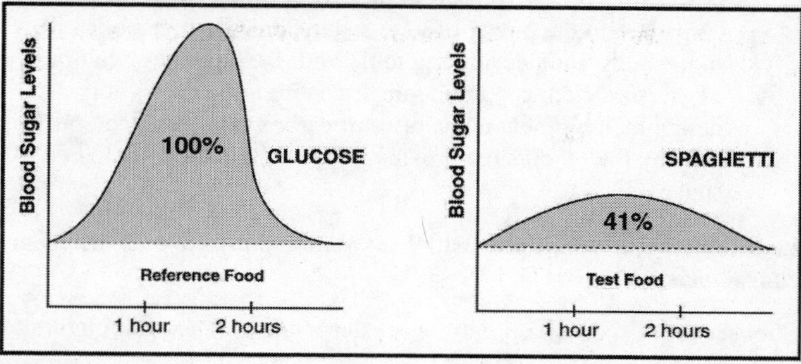

Diagram 3

Just to give you another example –

Let's say we are testing the GI of oranges-

We test oranges against the reference/standard food of pure sugar (glucose)

You ingest 3 tbsp pure sugar = 50grams pure carbohydrate.

You ingest an amount of oranges that will supply you with 50grams pure carbohydrate.

One orange contains 10grams of pure carbohydrate, so you need to eat 5 oranges to supply 50grams pure carbohydrate.

Your blood sugar response after eating 5 oranges is then compared to your blood sugar response after eating 3-tbsp sugar.

The GI of sugar = 100 and the GI of oranges = 44, meaning that oranges raise your blood sugar levels by only 44% of the amount that eating an equivalent amount of pure sugar carbohydrate does. So obviously its best to eat oranges rather than pure sugar, as the oranges will raise your blood sugar level less than sugar does.

The concept of the GI may be confusing to some, as when looking at a carbohydrate containing food we need to understand that there are 2 different characteristics of this food that are relevant to those trying to lose weight –

1) ***The total amount in grams of carbohydrate*** it contains, which determines its calorie content – eg. every gram of carbohydrate contains 4 calories. Too many calories can be fattening.

2) ***The GI of the carbohydrate*** food, which looks purely at the power of this type of food to raise your blood sugar levels, compared to the power of pure sugar. This is a metabolic effect in the body and has nothing to do with the amount or calories of this particular food that you are eating. The GI is not determined by the total calories or carbohydrate content, but only by the blood sugar raising power of this food compared to sugar.

Lets look at an example, which explains the above 2 different characteristics -

Choose foods containing an equivalent amount of carbohydrate *–for example*

Food	Carbohydrate (gms)	Calories	GI
Honey 1tbsp	17gms	68	58
Lima beans ½ cup	17gms	68	32

From the above you can see that 17grams carbohydrate = 68 calories = 1 tbsp honey = ½ cup Lima beans. So you may ask which is likely to be the most fattening food? Well they contain the same amount of carbohydrate and thus the same amount of calories, so they should be equally fattening – right?

Well not necessarily right!
The higher GI of the honey means that 1 tbsp of honey will raise your blood sugar more than ½ cup of Lima beans. This may not matter in those who are not overweight and do not suffer with Syndrome X.

However those with Syndrome X will find that the 1 tbsp of honey is more fattening than the ½ cup of Lima beans because the honey causes their blood sugar to rise more. This means that they will pump out more insulin, and we all know that insulin promotes the conversion of sugar into fat. So we are not just talking about grams of carbohydrate and calories, we are talking about the metabolic effect of carbohydrate foods in your body – that is what the GI is all about. As they say a calorie is not always just a calorie!

This may be all too confusing but the bottom line is -
If you are trying to choose between 2 foods that have equivalent amounts of carbohydrates – choose the one with the lower GI.

Foods that have a high GI raise your blood sugar levels higher and faster than foods that have a low GI.

Generally speaking for those people with Syndrome X, obesity or type 2 diabetes, it is far better to choose foods that have a low GI.

GI evaluation	GI VALUE
Low GI Foods	less than 55
Moderate GI Foods	56 to 70
High GI Foods	greater than 70

TABLE 4

Low GI foods are desirable because –
They do not cause the blood sugar levels to rise rapidly
They prevent high insulin levels and therefore the storage of fat
They are more filling and reduce hunger
They contain fibre, which reduces cholesterol levels

It has been shown that lowering the Glycaemic Index (GI) of the carbohydrates ingested (without changing the total amount of carbohydrate) improves blood sugar control by 10%. This is the same magnitude of improvement we see from treating type 2 diabetics with drugs to lower blood sugar.

The Glycaemic Index (GI) of foods is now Internationally recognised as being important in healthy food choices. The World Health Organisation (WHO) now recommends that people should choose foods that have a low GI.

In general eating low GI carbohydrates means that you will be eating far less processed foods, which will cut down your intake of sugar and hydrogenated vegetable oils. You will find low GI carbohydrate in foods such as legumes (beans, dried peas, lentils), whole gains such as oats, wheat, spelt, amaranth, barley, millet, brown rice, vegetables (except for potatoes, carrots & pumpkin) and many fruits.

Vegetable carbohydrates
Higher carbohydrate vegetables are potato, sweet potato, carrots, pumpkin and corn, although corn and sweet potato are lower than potatoes. Beetroot and peas contain carbohydrates, however normal serving sizes do not have a significant effect upon blood sugar levels. If starchy vegetables such as carrots, pumpkin and potatoes are eaten in normal serving sizes accompanied by protein, they will generally not

cause significant problems for those trying to lose weight. However you will find it easier to lose weight if you avoid the starchy vegetables during the first 6 weeks of the eating plan in this book – *see page 244.* Vegetables used for salads such as celery, tomatoes, cucumber, zucchini, leafy greens, lettuce, snow peas, onion, garlic, capsicum have very tiny amounts of carbohydrate and you can eat them freely.

Here are some ideas to help you swap from undesirable high GI foods to desirable low GI foods -

High GI Foods	Healthy Low GI Food Substitutes
Packaged snack foods such as cakes, muffins, bagels & cookies.	Biscuits/cakes made with whole grains & dried fruits, whole fruits, oats. A slice of whole grain bread.
White Rice (instant), Pastas made with refined flour	Long grain rice, brown rice, basmati rice, and lentils, beans and chickpeas
Tropical fruits such as bananas Kiwi, papaya & pineapple	Citrus fruits, apples, cherries, peaches, plums
Potato	New potatoes, legumes, corn, sweet potatoes, wholegrain pasta and rice
Packaged/processed breakfast cereals with added sugar	Home made or raw muesli made from oats, bran, nuts, seeds & psyllium with small amounts of dried fruits, cereals made with barley and oats
Breads especially white, but also some types of processed whole wheat Bread containing sugar	Sourdough, pumpernickel, stone ground wholemeal, or breads made with soy or baisen flour, grainy breads made with whole seeds
Packaged snack foods such as chips, pretzels, lollies	Raw nuts, seeds, avocado on Ryvita biscuits, small amounts dried apricots & peaches, any roasted legumes, Sandra Cabot's S-X snack pack.
Savoury biscuits (crackers) such as Salada, jatz	Water crackers, stone-ground crackers, Ryvita, Vita-weat crackers

The GI scale applies to carbohydrate foods, as foods mainly comprised of fat and/or protein do not raise the blood sugar levels significantly.

Some good low GI carbohydrates

Bread

Chapati

Chapati is flat Indian bread. The best type with the lowest GI of only 27 is made from chickpea flour also known as baisen flour.

Pumpernickel has a low GI of 51 and Sourdough bread has a low GI of 52. Stone ground breads such as whole-wheat stone-ground bread has a low GI of 53. In stone ground breads the entire grain is used and is a rich source of fibre, B vitamins and zinc.

Cereals

Oat bran and oatmeal of the old fashioned type (not instant) have a low GI of around 50.

Pearl barley has a very low GI of only 25. Pearl barley can be used as a breakfast cereal or in place of rice, and also added to soups or casseroles.

Bulgur is cracked wheat and has a GI of 48. Bulgur is used in "tabouli", which is a salad combination of onion, tomato, parsley and bulgur. Bulgur can also be used in vegetarian burgers, stews and casseroles or as a low GI cereal.

Rice bran has a very low GI of only 19. Rice bran can be added to breakfast cereals, muffins and cookies.

The GI of rice varies a lot depending upon the type of rice. The low GI varieties of rice are brown, Basmati and Japonica. Waxy or glutinous rice and Arborio rice have a higher GI.

Legumes

Beans of all varieties are generally low GI carbohydrates. Lentils and chickpeas are also healthy carbohydrates. In Asia soft blended lentils known as dhal (pronounced daal), provide a healthy low fat, low GI carbohydrate accompaniment to a meal. In Asia meat is expensive so it is common to include soybeans, tofu, dhal and many vegetables and seaweeds with the rice. This is a very healthy maintenance diet.

Soybeans and their products

Soybeans contain phytoestrogens known as isoflavones, which help to reduce the effect of excessive oestrogen levels. In peri-menopausal women who are overweight, excessive oestrogen levels may increase the risk of breast and uterine cancer, as well as causing weight gain around the hips and thighs. The phytoestrogens in soy products can help to reduce this oestrogen dominance.

I encourage you to eat soy products regularly (but not exclusively) by using the following –
Soybeans – canned or cooked
Okra – soybean pulp as a thickener
Soy flour – in baked goods
Tofu cubes – they can be marinated in garlic, chilli, ginger and sauces etc. and added to stir-fries. They can also be alternated with meat or chicken or seafood on a kebab.
Soymilk – can be used on cereals, in tea and coffee, including cappuccinos and in smoothies. Avoid soymilks with added sugar.
Soy nuts (roasted) - can be used in muesli, salads, or for snacks.
Soybeans and **tofu** are excellent very low GI carbohydrate accompaniments to meals. Soybeans are high in protein, omega – 3 fatty acids, fibre, minerals and B vitamins. Soybeans have a very low GI of only 18 and are excellent for those with Syndrome X.

Fruits

Apples are high in fibre and provide a low GI snack. The GI of a fresh raw apple is only 38. Apples contain a lot of fructose (fruit sugar), which is more slowly absorbed than glucose.
Dried apricots have a low GI of only 31 and make an excellent healthy snack, provided you do not eat too many at one sitting. Fresh apricots have a GI of around 57 and are high in the fruit sugar fructose. This contributes to their lower GI.
Oranges have a low GI of 44, are full of vitamin C, and make an excellent snack.
Fresh grapefruit has a low GI of only 25 and can be eaten with other fruits, or sprinkled with stevia, to temper their tart taste.
Fresh peaches have a low GI of 42 and make an excellent high fibre snack.
Fresh pears are high in fructose, which does not cause blood sugars to rise rapidly. They are good for a snack, with breakfast or for dessert. When fresh and raw their GI is only 38.
Fresh cherries are an excellent fruit for those with Syndrome X, as they have the lowest GI of any fruit. Cherries can be used widely with a GI index of only 22.
Plums are very nutritious with a low GI of 39.
Green Grapes are quite high in fruit acids, which contributes to their rather low GI of 46. They make a convenient snack especially with raw nuts.
Of all the tropical fruits, kiwi, mango and papaya have the lowest GI of between 50 and 60.

Grams of Carbohydrate and Glycaemic Index of foods

TABLE 5

Vegetables	Carbohydrates (gms)	GI
Asparagus (4 spears)	2.2	
Artichoke	12	
Alfalfa sprouts 100gms	3.0	
Avocado (peeled) 50gms	3.5	
Bamboo shoots 1 cup canned	4.0	
Bean sprouts 100gms	3.0	
Beans –green 25gms	2.0	
Broccoli 50gms	3.0	
Brussels sprouts (cooked) 100gms	4.0	
Cabbage –(cooked) 30gms	1.5	
Carrots 100gms	4.0	
Capsicum 40gms	2.0	
Cauliflower (cooked) 50gms	2.5	
Celery (1 stalk)	1.6	
Chives (raw) 2 tbs	1.0	
Sweet potato (1, baked)	37	54
Potato (one, baked)	33	93
New potato, small	28	62
Potato salad (1 cup)	33.5	
Corn sweet (1/2 cup, cooked)	20.6	55
Kale (1 cup, cooked)	6.7	
Spinach (1/2 cup, cooked)	3.4	
Winter squash 1 cup cooked	18.0	
Summer squash 1 cup cooked	8.0	
Cabbage (1 cup, cooked)	6.2	
Beans (green, cooked, 1 cup)	6.8	
Peas green (cooked, 1 cup)	19.4	48
Peas green (frozen) 1 cup	23.0	52
Cucumber (1cup, sliced, raw)	3.6	
Collard greens 1 cup	5.0	
Coleslaw (1 cup)	8.5	
Dandelion (1 cup)	6.7	
Mustard greens (1 cup, cooked)	5.6	
Kohlrabi (1 cup, cooked)	8.7	
Endive (1 cup)	2.1	
Pumpkin (1 cup, cooked)	20	75
Parsnips (1 cup, cooked)	23	97

Vegetables	Carbohydrates (gms)	GI
Radish 4 fresh	1.0	
Turnips (cooked, 1 cup)	11.3	
Tomato 1 small	5.0	38
Eggplant (cooked, ½ cup)	3.2	
Broccoli (1 cup, cooked)	8.5	
Pepper or capsicum(1 cup, raw)	7	
Onion (one tablespoon)	0.9	
Leeks ½ cup cooked	4.0	
Ginger ¼ cup raw	3.0	
Beets (cooked, ½ cup)	8.5	64
Carrots (1/2 cup, cooked)	8.2	90
Lettuce (one leaf)	0.4	
Cauliflower (1/2 cup, cooked)	2.9	
Mushrooms (1 cup)	3.1	
Parsley (1 tbs)	0.3	
Garlic (one clove)	1.0	
Water chestnuts canned 1 cup	17.0	
Zucchini 1 cup cooked	8.0	
Frozen vegetables 1 cup	24.0	
Fruits		
Tomato (1/2 cup)	2.9	
Tomato juice (1 cup)	10.4	
Strawberries 1/2 cup	5.3	
Apricots (one fresh)	4.6	42
Apricots dried 5 to 6 pieces	2.6	31
Nectarines 1	16.0	
Orange (1 medium)	16	44
Lemon (one)	6	
Banana (one)	26.6	55
Mango 1 cup	28	55
Mango – 1 whole	35	55
Honey dew melon (1/2 cup)	7.2	
Red & green grapes (1/2 cup)	7.9	
Pear –1	21	38
Avocado (1 medium)	20	57
Apple (1 medium)	20	38
Pineapple 1 cup fresh	21.2	66
Pineapple 2 slices fresh	10.0	66
Pineapple canned 1 cup	52.0	

Fruits	Carbohydrates (gms)	GI
Blueberries (1/2 cup)	11	
Raspberries (1/2 cup)	10.5	
Blackberries (1/2 cup)	9.2	
Cherries (1/2 cup)	10.2	23
Pink grapefruit ½	10.3	28
Grapefruit yellow ½	5.0	25
Grapes green 100gm	15.0	46
Lemon juice – 1cup	21.0	0
Plum 1 medium	9.0	29
Prunes one fresh	5.6	29
Peach 1 large	10.0	41
Peach dried 1 cup	98.0	
Peaches canned ½ cup	19.0	58
Papaya 1 medium	30.4	58
Kiwi (1 medium)	9	52
Olives - 4	trace	
Rockmelon ½ small	22.0	
Raisins 40gms	28.0	64
Raspberries 1 cup	14.0	
Rhubarb 1 cup	75.0	
Watermelon 1 cup	8.0	72
Dates 5	27.0	103
Figs 50gms	22.0	61

Legumes		
Soybeans (1/2 cup)	10.0	18
Tofu/bean curd (2 –inch cube)	2.9	
Tofu frozen dessert 60gms	21.0	115
Split peas ½ cup boiled	7	22
Navybeans (1 cup)	40.3	38
Lima (1 cup)	33.7	34
Black-eyed peas (1 cup)	38	42
Black beans ¾ cup	31	30
Baked beans canned ½ cup	24	48
Chana dal 1 & ½ cups	28	8
Lentils ½ cup boiled	16	28
Chickpeas boiled ½ cup	23	33
Chickpeas canned ½ cup	15	42
Red kidney ½ cup boiled	20	28
Red kidney beans canned ½ cup	19	52

Legumes	Carbohydrates (gms)	GI
Pinto beans dried ½ cup	22	38
Pinto beans canned ½ cup	18	44
Nuts and Seeds		
Peanuts (30gms)	5.4	15
Peanut butter natural - 1 tbsp	3.0	
Pumpkin seeds (30gms)	4.2	
Sunflower seeds (30gms)	5.6	
Sesame (1 tbsp)	1.4	
Walnuts (30gms)	4.2	
Pistachio (60gms)	14	
Almonds (30gms)	6.0	
Almond paste (30gms)	14.5	
Pecans (30gms)	4.1	
Brazil (30gms)	3.1	
Cashews (60gms)	18	
Macadamia (60gms)	10	
Coconut (30gms)	4.3	
Hazelnuts (30gms)	4.7	
Milk products		
Soy milk unsweetened – 1 cup	13	31
Whole milk 1 cup	11	27
Skim milk 1 cup	12	32
Chocolate milk 1 cup	26	
Cream (thick – 1 tbsp)	0.5	
Cream light – 1 tbsp	1.0	
Whipped cream 2 tbsp	1.0	
Cream (sour – 1 tbsp)	0.5	
Yogurt (plain – skim – 1 cup)	13	14
Yogurt (plain – whole – 1 cup)	12	
Yogurt fruit low fat – 1 cup	43	36
Ice cream ½ cup	15	61
Cheese		
Cheddar (30grams)	1.0	
Ricotta whole milk 1 cup	7.0	
Ricotta skim 1 cup	13	
Swiss 30grams	1.0	
Cottage skim – 1 cup	10	
Cottage whole – 1 cup	7	

Milk products	Carbohydrates (gms)	GI
Feta (30gms)	1.0	
Camembert (30gms)	0.5	
Grains and Cereals		
Noodles (cooked- 1 cup)	37.3	
Oatmeal cooked – 1 cup	25	45
Oat bran raw 1tbsp	7	55
Buckwheat ½ cup	20	54
Bulgur 2/3 cup	23	48
Couscous 2/3 cup	21	65
Corn flakes 1 & ¼ cups	24	84
Special K 1 cup	22	66
Muesli natural 2/3 cup	28	53
All bran ½ cup	22	42
Rice bran – 1 tbsp	5	19
Rice white cooked – 1 cup	50	72
Rice brown cooked 1 cup	37	55
Rice basmati 1 cup	50	58
Rice instant 1 cup	37	87
Rice (puffed – 1 cup)	11.5	82
Pearl barley ½ cup	22	25
Barley		25
Puffed wheat		80
Porridge		46
Shredded wheat		67
Pasta		
Spaghetti white		50
Spaghetti whole wheat		41
Macaroni		45
Fettuccini		32
Gnocchi		68
Star pastina		38
Vermicelli		35
Cellophane noodles		26
Breads		
Whole-wheat 1 slice	15	69
Bagel -1	36	
Bread crumbs 1 cup	73	

Breads	Carbohydrates (gms)	GI
Oat mix grain 1 slice	12	40
Pita 1 slice	33	57
Pumpernickel bread 1 slice	17	41
Rye 1 slice	15	62
Sourdough 1 slice	21	55
White bread 1 slice	21	70
Chapati (baisen) 1	25	27
Crackers		
Kavli – 2	16	71
Rice cakes – 3	123	82
Ryvita – 2	16	69
Water crackers – 3	18	78
Vita-weat – sandwich size –3	25	
Alcohol and Beverages		
Beer – 1 can	13	
Beer – light 1 can	5	
Spirits 45mls (a nip)	0	
Wine 100mls – 1 glass	3	
Coffee & tea no sugar	0	
Coffee & tea with sugar	22	
Cola 1 can	41	63
Fanta		68
Gatorade		78
Sugars		
Honey		60
Fructose (fruit sugar)		23
Maltose		110
Glucose		100
Lactose (milk sugar)		46
Animal protein (lean or fat, not fried in bread crumbs)		
Fresh or canned fish, red meat, pork, poultry, eggs	1 to trace amounts	
Oysters ½ cup	4	
Clams raw & canned 90gms	2	
Crabmeat canned 1 cup	2	
Fish sticks frozen 4	16	

Miscellaneous Items	Carbohydrates (gms)	GI
Tomato sauce 1 tbsp	4	
Tomato paste 1 cup	49.0	
Gherkin dill 1 medium	1.0	
Gherkin sweet 1 medium	5.0	
Relish or chutney 1 tbsp	5.0	
Cider vinegar 1 tbsp	1	
Garlic powder 1 tsp	2	
Onion powder 1 tsp	2	
Miso 30mls	8	
Cinnamon 1 tsp	2	
Curry powder 1 tsp	1	
Mustard powder 1 tsp	trace	
Oregano 1 tsp	1	
Paprika 1 tsp	1	
Black pepper 1 tsp	0.5	
Jam – fruit 1 tbsp	18	51
Soup – tomato canned 1 cup	33	38
Fast Food and Snack Food		
Cheese burger 1	28	
Fish burger 1	39	
Hamburger 1	20	
Pizza 1 slice	39	
Fried chicken ½ breast	13	
Roast chicken ½ breast	0	
Chocolate bar		69
Mars bar		75
Jelly beans		80
Potato chips		51
Oatmeal cookie with added sugar		54
Popcorn (popped – 1 cup)	5	55

Vegetables low in carbohydrates – Free foods

Alfalfa, asparagus, green beans, bamboo shoots, bean sprouts, cauliflower, cabbage, celery, collard greens, cucumber, dill pickle, eggplant, endive, fennel, kohlrabi, kale, lettuce, mushrooms, okra, onion up to 2 tbsp, parsley, capsicum, radish, spinach, ½ tomato, turnips, zucchini, water cress.

Vegetables and fruit servings under 5 grams of carbohydrates for those on a low carbohydrate diet –

½ avocado
blueberries 38 gms
strawberries 75gms
brussels sprouts 4
cabbage 90 gms
carrot – 1
eggplant 30gms
green beans 45gms
chilli pepper 1
spinach 60gms
tomato ½
waterchestnuts 4
Asparagus – 6 spears
broccoli 1 cup
cauliflower – 1 cup
cucumber – ½
leeks – ½ cup
mushrooms – ½ cup
parsley – ½ cup
capsicum – ½ cup
shallots – 1 tbsp

Meats and nuts contain only tiny amounts of carbohydrate, or none at all. Their GI is zero, and if eaten alone, they have negligible effects on blood sugar levels.

Vegetable and Seed Oils	
Flaxseed, canola, olive, sunflower, grapeseed etc) Butter Margarine Mayonnaise	All have 0 to trace amounts of carbohydrates

Note: The values above represent the average values taken from those in the scientific literature.

To search for Glycaemic Index of foods

There is a website designed by the University of Sydney called *www.glycemicbalance.com* which will enable you to calculate the Glycaemic Index of common foods.

12

Chapter Twelve

Sweeteners

Sweeteners

It seems that everyone's taste buds are getting sweeter. A report from the US Department of Agriculture shows a steady increase in the use of sweeteners with an increase from 56 kilograms per person in 1980 to 69 kilograms annually per person by 1999. Sugar consumption was only 5 ½ kilograms per person annually in the early 1800s.

It is normal for almost everyone to desire or even crave very sweet foods at different times during the day. These cravings can become particularly strong if we are highly stressed, our blood sugar is low, or if we have high levels of insulin (hyperinsulinaemia). Hormonal imbalances can also make us crave sugar during the pre-menstrual phase of the cycle, after childbirth and during menopause.

The worst type of sugar to eat is refined sugar, especially if it is combined with hydrogenated vegetable oils or saturated fat. Even so called "natural" sugar substitutes such as honey, raw sugar, molasses, barley malt, maple syrup, date sugar, etc. can be unhealthy if eaten in large amounts, as they can greatly elevate bloods sugar levels and thus insulin levels. These high insulin levels will hormonally direct the body to store fat.

It is always wise to use the most natural sweeteners available, as the body has enzyme systems that are able to absorb and digest natural foods. Artificial and chemically altered foods are difficult to metabolise and overwork the liver, and may produce harmful chemical waste products in the process. Over many years the safety or harmful effects of artificial and chemically altered sweeteners will become apparent.

Below we take a look at the various sugar substitutes that are available today for those who love the taste of "sweet".

The natural herbal sweetener called "Stevia" can be helpful for anyone who has a "sweet tooth", as it is very sweet but does not contain any calories and does not elevate blood sugar levels.

Refined sugar or table sugar is also known as sucrose. It contains 4 calories per gram. Sucrose causes a rapid rise in blood sugar and insulin levels, and is best avoided in those with Syndrome X.

Alternative Sweeteners to table sugar (sucrose)

These sugars are mainly nutritive sugars meaning that they contain calories.
Those marked with an * cause rapid elevations in the blood sugar and insulin levels in those with Syndrome X or diabetes.

Barley malt *
Honey *
Glucose *
Carmelized sugar *
Brown sugar *
Raw sugar *
Invert sugar (contains glucose and levulose) *
Dextrose *
Maltose *
Molasses *
Maple syrup and maple sugar *
Date sugar *
Fructo-oligosaccharides (FOS), which is safe for diabetics
Evaporated cane juice *
Rice syrup *
Corn syrup *
High fructose corn syrup (contains glucose and fructose) *
Liquorice root
Stevia, which is a natural herbal sweetener.

Fructose (crystalline) is a natural fruit sugar. It is 1.5 to 2 times sweeter than table sugar (sucrose), and thus smaller amounts can be used. Crystalline fructose can be used in cooking and baking and causes the baked product to brown faster. Although fructose contains 4 calories per gram (the same as sucrose) it does not cause such a large and rapid rise in blood sugar levels as sucrose does.

Sugar alcohols
Sugar alcohols are derived from sugar molecules but chemically are really alcohols. They vary in sweetness from as sweet as sugar to half as sweet as sugar. The better known sugar alcohols are xylitol, mannitol, sorbitol and lactitol. Sugar alcohols are also known as polyols and can be used as sugar substitutes by diabetics or those on a low-carbohydrate diet. They are not fully absorbed by the body but the amount that is absorbed can be used as energy without raising insulin

levels. Because they are incompletely absorbed from the gut they can produce a laxative effect if overused. They do contain calories but not as many calories as sugar. They are included in the total carbohydrate count on food labels. They are often used in sugar free chewing gum. Unfortunately sugar alcohols may trigger cravings for sugar and refined carbohydrates.

Artificial chemical sweeteners

Aspartame
Neotame
Saccharin
Cyclamates
Sucralose
Acesulfame - K

The glycaemic index (GI) of sugars and sweeteners can vary significantly. Many low GI sweeteners are mixed with high GI sweeteners as fillers. This is true if powdered sweeteners are mixed with fillers such as dextrose or maltodextrin. Although the addition of these high GI fillers does not usually change the calorie content greatly, it can affect the blood sugar levels if multiple packets of the sweetener are used over the day.

High GI sweeteners and sugars are often disguised in foods and appear on the label as such things as glucose polymers, dextrose, maltodextrins or invert sugar.

Saccharin
Saccharin was discovered in 1879 and is a zero-calorie sugar substitute that is approximately 300 times sweeter than sugar. Large amounts of saccharin have been shown to cause cancer in laboratory animals. So far human studies have not shown an increased risk of cancers in saccharin users although the long-term effect of saccharin in humans is still not known.

Sucralose
Sucralose is synthesised by chlorinating the sugar sucrose. Research has found that sucralose can cause many health problems in laboratory animals. At this time the long-term safety of sucralose in humans is unknown.

Aspartame

Aspartame was discovered in 1965 and is found in products such as Equal and Nutrasweet. Aspartame is comprised of methanol, phenylalanine and aspartic acid. Methanol is wood alcohol, which breaks down into formaldehyde in the body after ingestion. The FDA and the Dallas based Aspartame Consumer Safety Network have received thousands of consumer complaints about symptoms possibly related to aspartame use. Complaints have included headaches, seizures, depression, blurred vision and numerous neurological disorders. Dr Nuri Farber and Dr John Olney from the Washington University Medical School in St. Louis, Missouri believe aspartame is a suspicious causative factor in various health problems. The November 1996 edition of the Journal of Neuropathology and Experimental Neurology, contains their statement that "In the past two decades, brain tumour rates have risen in several industrialised countries, including the USA. Compared to other environmental factors putatively linked to brain tumours, the artificial sweetener aspartame is a promising candidate to explain the recent increase in incidence and degree of malignancy of brain tumours. Evidence potentially implicating aspartame includes an early animal study revealing a exceedingly high incidence of brain tumours in aspartame – fed rats, compared to no brain tumours in concurrent controls. We conclude that there is need for reassessing the carcinogenic potential of aspartame". (Olney, Farber, 1996). The FDA issued a statement in 1996 that "A recently published medical journal article raises the question whether any increased incidence in the number of persons with brain tumours in the USA is associated with the marketing of aspartame. Analysis of the National Cancer Institute's public database on cancer incidence in the USA does not support an association between the use of aspartame and the increased incidence of brain tumours. The FDA stands behind its original approval decision, but the agency remains ready to act if credible scientific evidence is presented to it." Despite this assurance from the FDA there are many researchers who do not agree with the FDA.

For more information visit - www.dorway.com
You can also E-mail Betty Martini at
Mission-Possible-USA@altavista.net from this site.

Betty is an activist who believes that aspartame should be banned and she can recommend several authoritative books on this subject. At this present time I believe that it is wise to avoid the artificial chemical aspartame as a sweetener, or foods which contain it.

The proponents of aspartame will tell you that it does not cause tooth decay and can help with weight control, however the natural sweetener Stevia also has these advantages.

Acesulfame

This artificial sweetener was approved by the FDA in 1988 and is a derivative of aceoacetic acid. This is a synthetic chemical, which is probably not metabolised by the body and is 200 times sweeter than sugar. The likelihood of long term danger in humans from this artificial chemical is currently unknown.

The long-term use of all the artificial chemical sweeteners has not been proven to be completely safe. I believe that substituting stevia for aspartame, acesulfame and saccharin is a safer alternative for those who wish to avoid sugar.

Stevia

Stevia is a safe non-caloric herbal sweetener.

Stevia is a sweetener extracted from a South American plant called Stevia Rebaudiana and has a very long history of worldwide use. Stevia leaves have been used to sweeten various teas by diabetic patients in Asian countries for many years, and no side effects have been observed.

The extraordinary sweetness of Stevia is due to a complex molecule called Stevioside, which is a glycoside that is composed of glucose, sophorose and steviol.

Stevia herb in its unprocessed form is very sweet being about 15 times sweeter than table sugar. Stevia extracts in the form of steviosides are hundreds of times sweeter then table sugar, ***so you only need tiny amounts.***

Different forms of Stevia

Stevia comes in different forms – leaves (fresh & dried), liquid, tablets and powder. The taste of Stevia can vary depending upon the brand name, and some brands will have a slight liquorice aftertaste while others will not. Stevia tastes slightly different from sugar and although pleasant in taste, it can be an acquired taste.

Stevia tablets

These can be dissolved in hot beverages like tea and coffee and are convenient to carry around in your purse. The amount can vary from ½ to 2 tablets per cup.

Stevia leaves

Fresh leaves

If you chew a leaf picked from a stevia plant you will experience a long-lasting very sweet taste that could be compared to liquorice. You may be able to buy some stevia cuttings and plant them in your garden or on the balcony. Stevia grows best outdoors in hot sunny climates. You can use the fresh leaves to sweeten your drinks.

Dried leaves

The dried leaf is a lot sweeter than a fresh leaf. If you add crushed dried leaves to tea or coffee you will need to adjust the amount to suit your palate – use very small amounts to begin with. Many people make the mistake of using too much stevia, and then complain about the flavour.

Dried stevia leaves can be used to sweeten –
Coffee and tea, spicy curries, sweet and sour stir-fries, sweet sauces and hot breakfast cereals.
Generally speaking 2 to 4 dried leaves are required. The dried leaves have more of an after taste than the other forms of stevia.

Stevia powder – green

The powder is produced by grinding dried leaves and is about 20 times sweeter than sugar. Although it can be added to drinks and hot dishes it has a stronger after taste than other forms of stevia. Generally speaking the white stevia extract powder, stevia tablets or clear liquid stevia are more pleasant with only a slight or negligible after taste.

Stevia powder – white

White stevia extract powder contains 90% of sweet glycosides and is around 300 times sweeter than sugar. It is the most popular form of stevia having the least after taste.

Liquid stevia concentrates

These liquid concentrates are made by mixing the white powder in distilled water, or grain alcohol. Usually only a few drops are needed to sweeten a cup of tea or coffee, a glass of home made lemonade or iced tea. They are found in health food stores and come in dropper-type bottles of various sizes.

Safety of Stevia

Stevia can be used as an alternative to artificial sweeteners and sugar in those with Syndrome X and type 2 diabetes.

According to research Stevia does not affect blood sugar levels and some studies show that Stevia may reduce blood sugar levels

Stevioside has been used safely among Indians in Paraguay and Brazil for over 200 years and also in Japan for over 20 years. It has been found to be safe and generally free of side effects and so far there has not been any reports of stevia plant toxicity.

A comprehensive study done at the Chulalongkorn University Primate Research Centre in Bangkok, Thailand (Yodyingyuad, 1991) examined the effects of stevioside in hamsters and their progeny. They tested 4 groups of 20 (one-month-old) hamsters that were equally divided amongst the sexes.

	1st group	2nd Group	3rd Group	4th Group (controls)
Daily dose of Stevioside In mg/ kg of hamster body weight	500mg/kg	1000mg/kg	2500mg/kg	zero

The above doses of stevia given to all 3 groups of hamsters are very large, considering that it would be unlikely that a person would use more than a total amount of 500 milligrams (mg) of stevia per day.

The above study showed that there was no significant difference in the growth of the first generation of hamsters receiving the various amounts of stevioside compared to the control group. The third generation of hamsters showed no significant differences in body weight, irrespective of the stevia doses used. The mating performance of three generations of hamsters receiving various doses of stevia was as good as the controls. There were no abnormalities in reproductive tissue samples of sperm and ovaries in hamsters given stevia. No abnormalities in growth or fertility could be demonstrated in hamsters of both sexes receiving these very high doses of stevia compared to controls. The designers of this study concluded, "The results of this study are astonishing. Stevioside at a dose as high as 2500mg per kilogram of body weight affects neither growth nor reproduction in hamsters. If this is true in other mammalian species including humans, this substance will be of great benefit to industry and medicine, and can be used more widely as a non-caloric sweetener in a variety of foods and drinks, as already seen in Japan and Brazil."

The 1997 June edition of Food and Chemical Toxicity published a paper titled "Assessment of the carcinogenicity of stevioside in rats." It discusses a study carried out by Dr. Toyoda from the National Institute of Health Sciences in Tokyo. Over two years, three groups of laboratory rats, equally divided among the sexes were tested.

	1st Group	**2nd Group**	**3rd Group (control group)**
Stevioside dose in percentage of daily diets	2.5%	5%	zero

After the two-year study was completed the surviving rats were euthanised. The organs of the rats were tested and almost no difference was found between the rats given stevia and the control rats. It was found that the female rats given stevioside had a lower incidence of breast tumours and the males had a lower incidence of kidney damage. The rats that received the stevioside weighed less than the rats in the control group. This is to be expected, as stevia does not contain any calories. Dr Toyoda and associates concluded, "Stevioside is not carcinogenic in rats under the experimental conditions described." If we look at an average person, the daily intake of stevioside could be estimated at the most, to be around 0.01% of the total daily food intake. The fact that rats given much higher amounts of stevia than this, did not experience an increased incidence of cancer is very positive.

In 1985 a study done at the College of Pharmacy, University of Illinois, Chicago looked at the effects of stevioside on a bacteria called Salmonella typhimurium. Although stevioside did not cause any toxic reactions, steviol, which is a breakdown product of stevioside, caused some DNA changes in this strain of bacteria. Of great significance is that these DNA changes occurred only in the presence of a liquid fraction made from the livers of rats who had been treated with the chemical called Aroclor 1254 and other chemicals. However no problems were found if steviol was given to the bacteria without first being exposed to the above chemical toxins. Thus this study has no significance to humans because their livers are not damaged by toxic chemicals before they ingest stevia. In 1993 researchers in the Dept of Biochemistry at Chiang Mai University, Thailand tested stevioside and steviol for mutagenicity (causing changes in DNA) in Salmonella typhurium bacteria and also in cultured human white blood cells. No mutations were caused by the stevioside even in high concentrations.

When a much higher dose was used weak mutagenicity was seen in the bacteria.

Of huge importance was the finding that no significant chromosomal effects/damage were produced in the human white blood cells from stevioside or steviol. The study concluded "stevioside and steviol are neither mutagenic nor clastogenic (able to damage chromosomes) in vitro (in test tube) at the limited doses." Adequate studies of stevia use during human pregnancy are not available and until properly performed, it is advisable to use stevia in only small amounts while trying to conceive and during pregnancy. We can assess the effect of substances in a test tube, on a bacteria or in a laboratory animal, but we cannot extrapolate from this its effect in the human body with 100% reliability. An assessment of all the studies published on stevia plus the long history of its safe consumption in several countries, reassures me that stevia is very safe for humans. This is particularly so because of the small doses of stevia required for use as an alternative to sugar

Stevia and Diabetes

Diabetics living in Asian countries have used stevia leaves with no side effects for many years. *(REF. 23)*

Some studies have shown that stevia extract may help to reduce excessive blood sugar levels. *(REF. 24)*

During 1986 scientists from the Universities of Maringa and Sao Paolo studied the effect of stevia on blood sugar levels. *(REF. 25)*

Five grams of stevia leaves in extract form were given to 16 healthy subjects every 6 hours, for 3 days. A GTT was done before and after the administration of the stevia extract. The results of the GTT were compared to those of another group of subjects that did not receive the stevia extract. In those with a predisposition to diabetes the GTT revealed a marked elevation of blood sugar levels. The subjects that received the stevia were found to have significantly lower blood sugar levels during the GTT. The outcome of this study gives a favourable indication that stevia can be beneficial to diabetics. Even if stevia by itself does not lower blood sugar levels, its use may allow diabetics to consume less sugar, which would be helpful in achieving better blood sugar control. At this time stevia's mode of action in lowering the blood sugar is not fully understood. A trial in the Department of Endocrinology and Metabolism at Aarhus University Hospital, Denmark, showed that stevioside improves insulin secretion from mouse pancreas in the presence of glucose. The researchers stated "Stevioside stimulates insulin secretion via a direct action on pancreatic beta cells. The results indicate that the compounds may have a potential role as an anti-hyperglycaemic agent in the treatment of type 2 diabetes mellitus"

Stevia in its pure form, whether it be called Stevia, Stevia extract, Stevioside, or Stevia concentrate, does not adversely affect blood levels of glucose or insulin, and may be used in those with Syndrome X

If you are diabetic your own doctor must guide you. There are references at the back of this book, which your doctor may wish to look up *(see page 341, 342).* You could begin to use stevia extract to sweeten your tea and coffee or lemonade and see how it affects your blood sugar levels. At the very least by using stevia you will be able to reduce your consumption of sugar and artificial sweeteners. We have also provided some stevia recipes that you may like to try.

Stevia and Weight Loss

Stevia is an exceptional aid to those trying to lose weight because it has ZERO CALORIES.

One ounce (28grams) of sugar contains 50 calories. One ounce of sugar is approximately 2 teaspoons of sugar and it is not uncommon for an average person to consume 360 grams (13 ounces) of sugar providing 650 calories every day. By replacing the sugar with stevia you will have a valuable aid to long term weight control.

Stevia will be used a lot as a sweetener in the future because extracts of pure stevia are hundreds of times sweeter than sugar.

Other advantages of Stevia

Research has shown that stevioside **does not cause tooth decay or tooth cavities.** This is because the substances in stevia that provide its sweetness do not ferment in the presence of bacteria. This is good news for children in whom the excessive consumption of sugar often leads to tooth decay and cavities.

In Japan stevia has been used for 20 years as a successful additive to products such as chewing gum, fizzy drinks, candies, and baked foods. In the near future we hope to see it used in the above ways in many more countries.

Several laboratory studies in rats showed that stevia is able to reduce blood pressure and provide a diuretic effect. *(REF. 26)*. A small study in Brazil studied 18 healthy human subjects who were given stevia leaf tea for 30 days. This study showed that stevia tea was able to effect a 10% lowering of pre-trial blood pressure levels. This is a small study and while the results are promising, more studies of stevia and its effects upon the human cardiovascular system are needed.

Some people using Stevia report improved digestion and less stomach upsets.

Stevia can be used as an anti-ageing tool. It is well known from numerous animal studies that reducing total calorie intake can extend life span. One of the factors contributing to ageing is the attachment of glucose to the proteins in the body, which is called the glycosylation of proteins. When glucose attaches to body proteins such as collagen and enzymes, damage to the proteins occurs causing cross-linking of proteins. These damaged proteins become less functional causing disturbances in cells and increasing degenerative diseases associated with ageing. With age the blood sugar levels tend to rise and so does the binding of glucose to our body proteins (glycosylation). This increases the hardening of arteries that supply our vital body organs with blood. Limiting the intake of calories and especially sugar can reduce the undesirable increase in glycosylation of body proteins typically seen with age. The use of stevia to reduce the intake of calories and sugar can only be helpful in preventing these physiological abnormalities of ageing.

Although the use of stevia as a therapeutic or medicinal substance has not as yet been fully investigated, we have observed a number of it's health promoting effects as discussed above.

How to use Stevia

Stevia can be used to completely replace added sugar in our diet. We can also use stevia with sugar, which will enable us to use less sugar, while still retaining the taste of sugar. We can combine stevia with honey, barley malt, rice syrup, molasses, raw brown sugar or fruit juices to reduce the amount of sugar in a recipe and our total consumption of sugar. Stevia extract can be used in recipes for baked foods, ice cream, puddings and smoothies. It can be added to freshly squeezed lemon juice or other citrus juices with a delicious result. Stevia is stable at high temperatures and thus can be used in hot dishes and baked foods. However baked foods made with stevia do not rise as much as those made with sugar. Stevia is not suitable as the sole sweetener in cakes or breads, which require yeast to rise. This is because sugar is needed to stimulate the rising properties of yeast. In such cases stevia can be used to replace half the sugar amount required in the recipe, with a big reduction in calories.

Baking or cooking stevia eliminates its after taste. The white stevia extract powder does not discolour food whereas the green stevia powder may slightly discolour food. Artificial sweeteners such as aspartame and saccharin have an obvious after taste and aspartame is unstable when heated.

It is important to realise that stevia extract is 300 times sweeter than sugar, and if you use excessive amounts this can result in excessive sweetness and after taste. It is best to start with tiny amounts of stevia until you find the amount that suits your palate as this can vary a lot between individuals. If you are overly sensitive to an after taste, mixing the stevia with a tiny amount of sugar or honey can eliminate this.

Conversion rates of Stevia and Sugar

Amount of Sugar	Equivalent amount of stevia extract powder	Equivalent amount of liquid stevia concentrate
1 teaspoon	a pinch to 1/16 teaspoon	2 to 4 drops, or one tablet
1 tablespoon	¼ teaspoon	6 to 9 drops or 3 tablets
1 cup	1 teaspoon	1 teaspoon

The above conversions are approximate for the following reasons –

- The sweetness may vary depending upon the brand of stevia used
- Sour or tart foods like lemons, grapefruits, limes, pineapple, green apples or cranberries need more stevia than naturally sweet foods like pears, ripe kiwi fruits or bananas.
- Personal taste – some like it sweeter than others

For more information on sweeteners call the Health Advisory Service on - 02 4655 8855 or visit www.sandracabot.com.

13

Chapter Thirteen

Dietary Fats

The good, the bad and the ugly

Dietary Fats – the good, the bad and the ugly

Most people struggling to lose weight avoid all dietary fats like the plague. Indeed they meticulously scour food labels to determine the fat content of foods. Fat has become a dirty word, probably because we know that it is a very calorie dense food providing 9 calories per gram of fat.

We know that it is not just the amount of calories that you consume that makes you fat – it is just as important to choose the source of the calories wisely. Some dietary fat is good for you, and a blanket ban on all dietary fat means that we throw out the good fats along with the bad fats.

Dietary fat does not cause blood insulin levels to rise significantly, so you do not have such high amounts of the fat producing hormone insulin in your body. Dietary fat is not converted to glucose as easily as dietary protein, which is one of the reasons why dietary fat does not elevate insulin levels significantly.

In those who eat no fat, there can be health problems as fat is an essential dietary item. Without any dietary fat your metabolic rate will slow down so that you burn calories less efficiently. This is because the cells and their tiny internal organs are made of essential fatty acids. If you do not get enough dietary essential fats, your cells will suffer, and their membranes and internal organs will be of inferior structural quality. The cells will not function efficiently and will not produce enough cellular energy, resulting in fatigue and a sluggish metabolism. These things will make you fatter when you start to eat normally. Essential fatty acids make your cell membrane walls softer, so that nutritional substances such as carnitine are able to take fat out of the cell. Californian endocrinologist Dr Diana Schwarzbein has been researching dietary fat intake for more than ten years. She has found that low fat diets are always followed by a decline in health. Indeed her research of hundreds of women found that low-fat fanatics eventually increase body fat and may have increased blood pressure.

Your body cannot manufacture its own essential fats, and that is why we say they are essential to obtain from your diet.

Many people on a low fat diet become yoyo dieters, and as they lose weight their metabolism slows down. When they come off the low fat diet and start to eat "normally" again, their slow metabolism cannot cope with the increased calories and they put on more weight than before they started the diet.

We now know that the low-fat message given to us since the 1970s was too simplistic. We know that low fat diets do not work – just look at the USA, where people have access to more processed no-fat or low-fat foods than any other country, and yet there is an epidemic of obesity and diabetes!

Dietary fat is used to make essential body hormones. Sex hormones and cortisone are made from the fat cholesterol, and if you do not eat any cholesterol, your liver will make enough cholesterol for your body to use for making steroid hormones. Cholesterol is also used to make cell membranes and the insulating sheaths around nerve fibres. The fat cholesterol is essential in the body for good health.

In my eating program you will get healthy amounts of cholesterol in your diet.

In the past, people have been wrongly educated to avoid foods containing cholesterol such as eggs and shellfish for fear that these foods may raise blood cholesterol levels. We now know that cholesterol is essential in the human body, and that a healthy liver can adjust its production of cholesterol to compensate for increased dietary consumption of cholesterol. If your liver is healthy it will manufacture the good cholesterol called HDL cholesterol, which prevents atherosclerosis. If your liver is unhealthy and fatty, it will manufacture excessive amounts of the bad LDL cholesterol, even if you follow a low fat diet.

Statistics show that almost 50% of men and 39% of Australian women over the age of 20 have total cholesterol levels that are above the desirable range (defined as above 5.0 millimoles per litre). This does not mean that much by itself, as it is more important to know if the total cholesterol is comprised largely of the good HDL or the bad LDL cholesterol. Many of these people do not eat large amounts of saturated fat and their problem comes from eating too much refined carbohydrate, processed hydrogenated oils and a sluggish liver.

In a small percentage of the population there exists an inherited defect called “familial hypercholesterolaemia”, which results in grossly elevated cholesterol levels and sometimes triglyceride levels. In these people there is a genetic impairment of the liver’s ability to regulate cholesterol production, and it is necessary to reduce cholesterol foods and take cholesterol-lowering medication.

So the good news is that the vast majority of people can eat and enjoy a moderate amount of cholesterol containing foods.

Essential fatty acids are used to manufacture vital body hormones called prostaglandins and eicosanoids, which transmit messages between body cells and also exert an anti-inflammatory effect. Those with a dietary deficiency of essential fatty acids can suffer serious health problems. Fats are needed for the healthy appearance of the hair and skin, so those on very low fat diets often look drawn, with a "dried out look" and lifeless dry hair.

The metabolic effect in the body of the food you eat is just as important as the calories it contains. So eating fat is OK, as long as you abide by some simple rules –

- You cannot eat unlimited amounts of fat, as it is high in calories.
- You should choose the good fats and avoid the bad fats, as the latter will slow down your metabolism and increase the risk of a fatty liver.

Understanding dietary fats

Fats are made up of carbon and hydrogen atoms. The carbon atoms form the chain or backbone of the fat, and are attached to hydrogen atoms at the sides, with some oxygen attached at the end of the chain. If the carbon atoms are attached to the maximum number of hydrogen atoms they can hold, the fat is called saturated fat.

If the carbon atom chains are missing some hydrogen atoms, the carbon atoms form double links (bonds) with other carbon atoms to fill up the gaps. These types of fats are called unsaturated, as they are not saturated with hydrogen atoms.

Unsaturated fats may be mono-unsaturated, meaning that they have one extra carbon double bond, or poly-unsaturated meaning they have 2 or more double carbon bonds.

Examples of saturated fats are butter, lard, animal fats, and some vegetable fats such as palm oil and coconut oil. Saturated fats are usually solid at room temperature.

Unsaturated fats such as seed and vegetable oils like olive oil, canola oil, and flaxseed oil, are liquid at room temperature. Corn oil and safflower oil are very high in polyunsaturated fats, whilst olive oil and nut oils are high in mono-unsaturated fats.

Animal fats are saturated and contain cholesterol, whereas plant foods, apart from coconut and palm oil, usually do not contain cholesterol.

The conventional dietary philosophy of today tells us to avoid cholesterol, as it will block our arteries with plaque, and instead we are told to eat a lot of polyunsaturated fat, which we are told will keep our arteries free of plaque. Many people follow this theory and use loads of margarine and cheap processed polyunsaturated fats, but we still have a very high incidence of heart disease, strokes and obesity in our fat conscious society. A presentation by Dr Tirshwell at the 1999 AHA Conference reported the findings of a study, which looked at the cholesterol levels of stroke victims compared to cholesterol levels amongst healthy subjects. Surprisingly it showed that brain haemorrhages were significantly more common in subjects with low cholesterol. *(REF. 27)*

Another study looked at a group of men who first ate a moderately high fat diet followed by a low fat diet. During the low fat diet phase of the trial, around one third of the men developed undesirable changes in their blood fat profile. In particular, their triglycerides and LDL cholesterol went up, and their good HDL cholesterol went down. *(REF. 28)*

You see its not as simple as avoiding saturated fats and replacing them with polyunsaturated fats – it's the quality of the fats that we eat that is so important. We need to avoid processed hydrogenated fats, deep fried foods, and fats that are oxidised (not fresh).

What we need is not so much a low fat diet, we need the right fat diet!

The right fats – healthy fats

These are generally known as the essential fatty acids (efa's), because they are essential to get in the diet, and are essential for good health. Because our food has become increasingly processed and many people erroneously follow low fat diets, I have found that deficiencies of essential fatty acids are very common. Your liver can manufacture cholesterol, but it cannot manufacture the essential fatty acids (efa's).

From the two essential fatty acids – known as omega 3 and omega 6 efa's, your body needs to make twenty different fatty acids, which are vital to good health.

Omega 3 fatty acid is also known as linolenic acid.
Omega 6 fatty acid is also known as linoleic acid.

Good sources of omega 3 efa's are –

Egg yolks, especially the omega – 3 enriched eggs
Nuts, especially walnuts and walnut oil (great on salad dressing)
Flaxseeds and their cold pressed oil
Cold water fish such as mackerel, cod, herring, tuna, salmon and sardines
Fish oil
Canola oil (cold pressed)
Soybeans
The leaves and seeds of most plants

Good sources of omega 6 efa's are –

Evening primrose oil
Borage seed oil (starflower oil)
Blackcurrant seed oil
Egg yolks
Dark green leafy vegetables
Seeds – sesame seeds, pumpkin seeds, sunflower & safflower etc
Whole grains

Good sources of omega 9 efa's –

These are not essential in the diet, but still they have great health advantages for metabolism and the immune system. Omega 9 efa's are also known as oleic acid. Omega 9 efa's are high in –
Olives and olive oil
Avocados and avocado oil
Nut oils including peanut oil
Sesame oil

Increase the essential fatty acids in your diet

We need to be specific here because many people believe that they get enough efa's by consuming cooking oils, which are relatively cheap and available in plastic containers on super market shelves. These commercial oils have been processed with chemicals at high temperatures, which damages their original essential fatty acids.

I strongly encourage you to buy only the good quality, cold pressed, unprocessed, unrefined oils that are usually available in glass containers or bottles of a darker colour than transparent plastic. Essential fatty acids are very fragile and are easily damaged and oxidised by exposure to heat, air and light. To protect them in their original form it is best to buy them and keep them in opaque containers in the refrigerator. You must protect your oils if you want them to protect you.

Olive or palm oils are best for high temperature cooking such as stir fries or sauteing. Do not cook with flaxseed oil or indeed heat it in any way, as you will damage and oxidise its fragile omega efa's.

Healthy ways to increase your consumption of efa's

- Eat **nuts** such as walnuts, pecans, Brazil, almonds, macadamias, hazelnuts, cashews, and peanuts. When it comes to peanut butters buy only the natural types, as many commercial smooth peanut butters are contaminated with large amounts of sugar and transfatty acids.

- **Salad dressings** are a good way of increasing your intake of beneficial efa's. Mayonnaise (dairy free), cold pressed oils, such as olive oil and flaxseed, nut oils, avocado oil, and lemon, and apple cider vinegar are healthful ways to increase the nutritional value of your salads. Flaxseed oil is nice to add to your salads or dry baked vegetables as it has a very mild, almost flavourless taste, and is a very rich source of omega 3 fatty acids. Do not use the cheap processed mostly polyunsaturated cooking oils for salad dressings. Replace them with unrefined cold pressed virgin olive oil, flaxseed oil and other cold pressed vegetable oils that are mostly mono-unsaturated or high in omega 3 fatty acids. We need to eat a lot of salads to keep our liver healthy, so the salad dressings will be a regular source of efa's in our diet. Many fat – free salad dressings are unhealthy, being loaded with sugar and chemicals and do not taste that great – indeed they are bad enough to put you off eating salads!

- **Spreads** – tahini, humus, nut spreads (unprocessed), avocadoes, olive oil

- Start to eat **fish** regularly, especially the cold water fish like tuna, salmon, cod, sardines, mackerel, herring and blue fish. Eating fish regularly can greatly reduce your risk of sudden cardiac death. *(REF. 29)* The omega 3 efa's in fish and fish oil, act as natural anti-inflammatory substances, and it is well known that fish oil can help those with auto-immune diseases, asthma and skin disorders such as eczema and psoriasis.

- **Eggs** are an excellent source of efa's and complete protein. Eggs are also an excellent source of the sulphur bearing amino acids, which are needed by the liver. Do not worry about the cholesterol, as provided the eggs are fresh and you do not fry them, the cholesterol in eggs will not harm you. Some dietary cholesterol is good for you, and if you do not eat any cholesterol, your liver will manufacture this vital fat.

- Eat plenty of **dark green leafy vegetables** and avocados and some eggplant to increase the healthful efa's. You can steam dark green leafy vegetables or stir-fry them, juice them or eat them raw in salads.

Benefits of the omega –3 fatty acids –
Reduction of heart disease
Reduction of blood clotting
Reduction of insulin resistance
Reduction of the risk of diabetes
Reduction of the risk of irregular heart beats, which is a common cause of sudden death after a heart attack.

The balance of omega 6 efa's to omega 3 efa's should be approx 2:1
In general the average Australian consumes too much omega 6 fatty acid compared to omega 3 fatty acids. This is because we consume excess amounts of cheap processed refined oils made from soy, canola, safflower and corn, which are very high in omega 6 efa's and relatively deficient in omega 3 efa's. We do not eat sufficient amounts of foods high in the omega 3 efa's such as fish, nuts, nut oils, seeds, whole grains, unrefined cold pressed vegetable oils and egg yolks. This imbalance of omega 6 to omega 3 efa's combined with the over consumption of transfatty acids found in margarine and many snack foods, partially explains why in this day and age we have such high levels of heart disease, and inflammatory diseases.

Transfatty acids – the really ugly fats!

Transfatty acids are man made fats that originate from vegetable oils. Most margarines are the best known examples, and are processed by taking a vegetable oil, removing the essential fatty acids, and forcing additional hydrogen atoms into the carbon chain. That's why these oils are called partially hydrogenated vegetable oils. This hydrogenation process makes the fat more saturated, which means it is solid, albeit a soft solid, at room temperature. Thus it is easy to spread and is convenient.

It's a pity that it is convenient, because transfatty acids and other partially hydrogenated vegetable oils are totally unnatural – we could even say they are alien to the body, as our cells find it very hard to use them. You could call trans-fatty acids social misfits in cellular society. Indeed our cells do not know what to do with trans-fatty acids – they not only block the use of the natural unprocessed efa's that you eat, they end up being deposited into your cell membranes. The problem is that they do not fit the cell membranes because they are the wrong shapes, so you end up with weakened cell membranes with holes in them.

The liver does not know how to utilise transfatty acids efficiently either and they may accumulate in the liver causing a fatty liver, especially if you eat them with a lot of refined carbohydrates.

Transfatty acids also cause your body to secrete more insulin than normal after a glucose load. This is another reason they cause weight gain. *(REF. 30)*

Transfatty acids have a very adverse effect upon your blood fats – they cause an elevation of undesirable LDL cholesterol, triglycerides and lipoprotein(a), and lower your good HDL cholesterol. This disturbance of blood fats is a potent predictor of cardiovascular disease.*(REF. 30)*

Studies showing the dangers of transfatty acids first appeared in the 1950s. Margarine was first developed as a cheap substitute for butter around 1910. Heart disease and obesity were uncommon early in the 20th century, before the introduction of trans fatty acids.

The huge Nurse's Health Study has shown that the risk of heart disease is nearly double if you get just 2% of your calories from transfatty acids. According to many researchers, including fat expert Mary Enig, many people get around 4% of their daily calories from transfatty acids. *(REF. 31)*

Whilst everyone is blaming our high incidence of obesity and cardiovascular disease upon animal fats and cholesterol, we should take a very careful look at the man made transfatty acids.

Sources of the transfatty acids are -

- Many margarines are high in transfatty acids.
- Foods deep-fried in polyunsaturated vegetable oils such as chips and batter. When you deep-fry any foods in sunflower, corn and other vegetable oils, you will cause the production of unhealthy trans-fatty acids. It is healthier and less fattening to fry foods in saturated fats such as palm or coconut oil, which are more stable, and not as easily damaged by extreme temperatures. I do not recommend that you eat deep fried food regularly, but if you eat it for a special treat, use the saturated palm or coconut oils, and not the cheap polyunsaturated vegetable cooking oils. Many of the fat-vats in fast food places contain fats that are continually reused – they are repeatedly heated, exposed to the air and light and become highly oxidised – this is a potent source of oxidised fat and free

radicals. Even saturated oils like lard, palm and coconut oils should not be re-used or reheated. A large serve of deep fried chips at a take-away restaurant could contain around 6 grams of transfatty acids.

- Potato chips in packets – they may state they are cholesterol free, but so what, the cholesterol is not the enemy!
- Many fast foods.
- Many baked and packaged foods – biscuits, cookies, cakes, buns, breads, doughnuts and muffins, etc.
- Many prepared foods such as - mayonnaise, salad dressings, dips and spreads, etc.
- Many brands of candy bars and snack bars.

14

CHAPTER FOURTEEN

Food Labels

How to read and assess them

Food Labels

Have you ever been in the Supermarket or health food store and seen people pouring over food labels? I bet you have! It seems to have become of more interest to people today to read about what they are putting into their mouths. Then again you may have looked at these people and thought that they were eccentric – after all in the busy rush and tear of life who has time for that type of obsession?

Well its really not that hard to understand a food label in a general way that will help you to make better food choices.

Be aware of what to look for and what to avoid on food labels. Avoid foods that have labels stating the presence of white flour, cornstarch, corn syrup, dextrose, maltose, fructose, lactose, sorbitol, aspartame, added sugar and hydrogenated vegetable oils.

Many Supermarkets have health food sections, which is great to see, but even some so called health foods can be full of the bad fats and added sugar.

• Let us take a look at a basic food label – in this case it is from a brand of creamy peanut paste.

Creamy Peanut Butter (Brand A)	
Nutrition Facts Serving size 2 tbs (32gm) Servings per package 35	
Amount Per serving	
Calories 200 Calories from fat 140	
	% Daily value
Total Fat 16g	25%
Saturated fat 3g	15%
Cholesterol 0mg	0
Sodium 140mg	6%
Total Carbohydrate 6g	2%
Dietary fibre 2g	8%
Sugars 3g	
Protein 7g	
Ingredients: peanuts, sugar, hydrogenated vegetable oil (cotton seed & rapeseed), molasses, salt and diglycerides.	

The peanut butter **(Brand A)** is not recommended for your good health. How can you tell this from the label? The only clue is to read the ingredients, which states that it contains added sugar and hydrogenated vegetable oils. These are the oils you want to avoid, as they are processed oils laden with man made transfatty acids.

• Now let us take a look at the label from a healthy natural creamy peanut butter and see if you can spot the differences!

Creamy 100% Natural Peanut Butter (Brand B)	
Nutrition Facts Serving size 2 tbs (32gm) Servings about 14	
Amount Per serving	
Calories 200 Calories from fat 150	
	% Daily value
Total Fat 16g	25%
Saturated fat 2.5g	13%
Cholesterol 0mg	0
Sodium 110mg	5%
Total Carbohydrate 7g	2%
Dietary fibre 2g	9%
Sugars 2g	
Protein 7g	
Ingredients: peanuts	

Comment: There are minor insignificant differences between the two Nutrition Facts panels, on Brand A and Brand B, which would not help you to decide which brand of peanut butter to buy. It is the ingredients list that will make the decision for you – in Brand B the only ingredients are real natural roasted peanuts and nothing else – there is no added sugar and no hydrogenated oils – in other words there is none of the unhealthy transfatty acids. So if you were "switched on", you would buy Brand B and help your liver!

• Now lets compare three different brands of salad dressings, to discover which is best for those with Syndrome X and weight excess.

Creamy Salad Dressing (Brand A)	
Nutrition Facts Serving size 2 tbs (29gm) Servings 24	
Amount Per serving	
Calories 150 Calories from fat 140	
	% Daily value
Total Fat 16g	25%
Saturated fat 2.5g	13%
Cholesterol 10mg	3%
Sodium 290mg	12%
Total Carbohydrate 1g	0%
Dietary fibre 0g	0%
Sugars 1g	
Protein 0g	
Ingredients: hydrogenated soybean oil, sugar, vinegar, egg yolks, salt, skim milk, garlic juice, natural buttermilk flavour, monosodium glutamate, preservatives, spice, dried parsley, lemon juice concentrate, natural flavour.	

Raspberry Fat Free Salad Dressing (Brand B)	
Nutrition Facts Serving size 2 tbs (30ml) Servings 8	
Amount Per serving	
Calories 35 Calories from fat 0	
	% Daily value
Total Fat 0g	0%
Saturated fat 0g	0%
Cholesterol 0mg	0%
Sodium 180mg	7%

Total Carbohydrate 9g	3%
Dietary fibre 0g	0%
Sugars 8g	
Protein 0g	

Ingredients: water, high fructose corn syrup, apple cider vinegar, cucumber juice, raspberry concentrate, lemon juice concentrate, salt, dehydrated red bell peppers, Hibiscus fruit extract, citric acid, garlic powder, onion powder, xanthan gum, preservative, natural flavour.

Extra Virgin Olive Oil Cold pressed (Brand C)	
Nutrition Facts Serving size: 1 tbs (15ml) Servings: about 66	
Amount Per serving	
Calories 120 Calories from fat 120	
	% Daily value
Total Fat 14g	22%
Saturated fat 2g	10%
Cholesterol 0mg	0%
Sodium 0mg	0%
Total Carbohydrate 0g	0%
Dietary fibre 0g	0%
Sugars 0g	
Protein 0g	
Ingredients: cold pressed virgin olive oil	

Comment: Brand A of the salad dressing contains hydrogenated soybean oil, which contains unhealthy transfatty acids. It also contains added sugar and monosodium glutamate, which can cause headaches in some people.
Brand B of salad dressing is low in calories but contains a lot of added sugar from high fructose corn syrup. This will cause blood sugar to rise thus stimulating an increase in insulin levels.
Brand C of salad dressing is lower in calories than Brand A, and is free of hydrogenated transfatty acids and is free of added sugar. It will have no effect upon blood glucose or insulin levels, and provides valuable mono-unsaturated fatty acids. Brand C is the preferred salad dressing for those with Syndrome X.

• Now lets look at the label of a very popular brand of breakfast cereal

Crunchy Wheat & Rice flakes with strawberries (Brand A)	
Fat Free!	
Nutrition Facts Serving size 1 cup (31gm/1.1oz) Servings: about 11	
Amount Per serving	
Calories 110 Calories from fat 0	
	% Daily value
Total Fat 0g	0%
Saturated fat 0g	0%
Cholesterol 0mg	0%
Sodium 220mg	9%
Potassium 75mg	2%
Total Carbohydrate 25g	8%
Dietary fibre 1g	4%
Sugars 10g	
Other carbohydrates 14g	
Protein 4g	
Ingredients: rice, sugar, and whole grain wheat, wheat gluten, freeze dried strawberries, defatted wheat germ, non-fat dried milk, high fructose corn syrup, salt, wheat flour, malt flavouring.	

Comment: Cereal "Brand A" may well be fat free as they have stripped all the good fats from the wheat germ, and destroyed its vitamin E content in the process. You will note that its main ingredient is carbohydrate, which is in good part derived from refined sugar and refined high fructose corn syrup. This breakfast cereal is highly processed, and will cause a rapid rise in blood sugar, which is not the way to start your day if you have Syndrome X. You are better off to choose unrefined cereals, (such as muesli) with no added sugar or corn syrup, and you will not have the rapid rise in blood sugar after breakfast.

• Now lets look at some Premium chocolate chip cookies

Chocolate Chip Premium Cookies (Brand A)	
Nutrition Facts Serving size 1 cookie (35gm) Servings 26	
Amount Per serving	
Calories 150 Calories from fat 70	
	% Daily value
Total Fat 7g	11%
Saturated fat 4g	21%
Cholesterol 10mg	4%
Sodium 95mg	4%
Total Carbohydrate 22g	7%
Dietary fibre < 1g	4%
Sugars 15g	
Protein 1g	
Ingredients: chocolate chips, bleached wheat flower, sugar, butter, margarine (partially hydrogenated vegetable oils from soybean & cottonseed) salt, diglycerides, artificial flavour, eggs, fructose, polydextrose, high fructose corn syrup, Corn syrup, salt, baking soda, coconut oil, and numerous preservatives	

Comment: "Brand A" cookies are loaded with refined sugars and hydrogenated vegetable oils (transfatty acids). These things will send your blood glucose soaring along with your insulin levels.

The transfatty acids will be difficult for your liver to process and will adversely affect your blood fats.

I suggest that you try to find some healthy cookies free of added refined sugar and transfatty acids.

• Now lets look at some healthy bread

Sprouted Rye Bread - Totally Natural **(Brand A)**	
Nutrition Facts Serving size 1 slice (34gm) Servings 20	
Amount Per serving	
Calories 60 Calories from fat 10	
	% Daily value
Total Fat 1g	2%
Saturated fat 0g	0%
Cholesterol 0mg	0%
Sodium 150mg	6%
Total Carbohydrate 11g	4%
Dietary fibre 2g	8%
Sugars 1g	
Protein 3g	
Ingredients: Organically grown sprouted wheat berries, sprouted whole rye, molasses, wheat gluten, fresh yeast, sunflower seeds, poppy seeds, salt, soy lecithin, sesame seeds, dill weed, caraway seeds, celery seeds	

• Now lets look at another bread

Wheat Premium Bread (Brand B)	
Nutrition Facts Serving size 1 slice (32gm) Servings 21	
Amount Per serving	
Calories 90 Calories from fat 30	
	% Daily value
Total Fat 3g	5%
Saturated fat 0g	0%
Cholesterol 0mg	0%
Sodium 115mg	5%
Total Carbohydrate 14g	5%
Dietary fibre 2g	8%
Sugars 3g	
Protein 4g	
Ingredients: cracked wheat, water, sunflower seeds, sugar, wheat gluten, walnuts, partially hydrogenated soy bean oil, yeast, salt, barley, wheat starch, rye, malt, corn, syrup, soy lecithin, millet, oats, diglycerides, brown rice, wheat flour.	

Comment: Brand A - bread is very good and has a small amount of unrefined sugar in the form of molasses. Brand B - bread has got quite a lot of good ingredients but it is spoilt by the addition of refined sugar and hydrogenated soybean oil (transfatty acids). So you can see that you really need to look at the ingredients list to choose the most suitable food for your health.

Vegetable Chicken Burger – (Brand A)	
Nutrition Facts Serving size 1 patty (85gm) Servings 2 per container	
Amount Per serving	
Calories 120 Calories from fat 30	
	% Daily value
Total Fat 3g	5%
Saturated fat 0g	0%
Cholesterol 0mg	0%
Sodium 390mg	16%
Total Carbohydrate 6g	2%
Dietary fibre 3g	10%
Sugars 1g	
Protein 17g	22%
Ingredients: water, textured soy protein, wheat gluten, cold pressed canola oil (non – GMO), natural flavour from vegetable sources, yeast extract, carrageenan , salt, vegetable gum, onion powder, organic cane juice, lemon juice powder, potato starch, konjac flour, garlic powder, spices, paprika	

Comment: "Brand A" vegetable "make believe chicken burger" is basically quite healthy and is suitable for vegetarians with Syndrome X. It is very low in carbohydrate, does not contain added refined sugar, and is free of trans-fatty acids. It is free of trans-fatty acids because the canola oil is cold pressed. Although it does not contain any chicken or meat, it is high in protein. This food will not cause large elevations of blood sugar or insulin levels. It is free of artificial chemicals and preservatives.

15

Chapter Fifteen

Body Types and Weight Gain

Body Types and Weight Gain

There are four classic body shapes or body types – they are the Android, the Gynaeoid, the Thyroid and the Lymphatic body types. They are classified according to their shape or anatomical proportions. The four Body Types have unique hormonal and metabolic characteristics, which explains why some body types gain weight easily and are more prone to cellulite. Your body type also determines the areas of your body where excess fat will accumulate.

The vast majority of people will belong to one of these four body types. Around 10% of people are a combination of two body types. The body types are genetically determined so you will probably find someone in your own family with the same body type as yourself. Your body type determines your metabolic type and is important to know because it explains the foods that may cause problems for you. When you avoid the foods that are incompatible with your body type weight loss becomes much easier.

Android Body Type

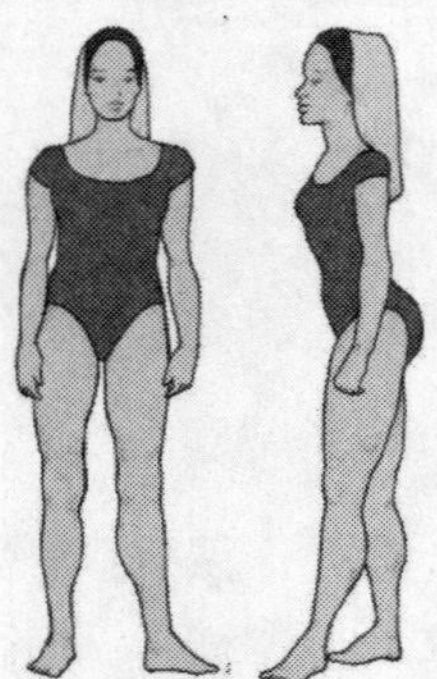

Android Ideal

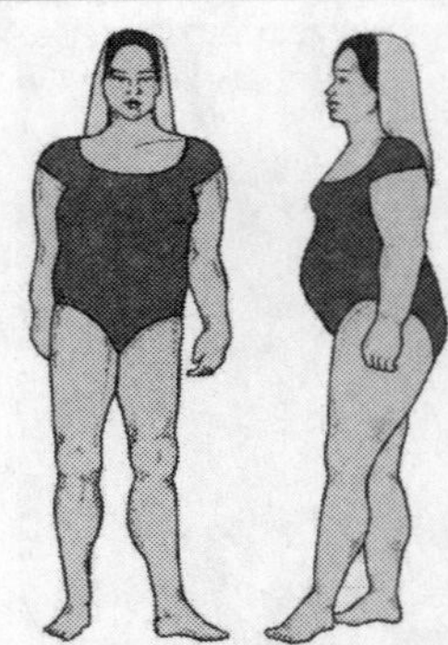

Android Overweight

Approximately 40% of women (and most men) belong to this body type, which is characterised by broad shoulders, strong muscular arms and legs, a narrow pelvis and narrow hips. The waistline does not curve inwards very much, so the trunk has a somewhat straight up and down appearance. Android women have a "boyish figure", and are usually good at sports and are strong, energetic and healthy. Android shaped persons are often very strong and able to work long hours in physical occupations.

Android-shaped people have an anabolic metabolism, which leads to a body building tendency in the upper part of the body.

They tend to produce more male hormones than do other body types, which adds to the body building tendency. Weight gain occurs in the upper part of the body and on the front of the abdomen, so that an apple-shape may develop.

Android persons tend to crave salty, savoury foods and carbohydrates.

If Android people gain a lot of weight they tend to become "apple shaped" – *see page 174*

Protein is good for Androids, but it should be low fat protein, such as very lean red meats and seafood. Android women should consume foods high in plant hormones, as this will give their hormones a more feminine pattern. Plant hormones are found in all plant foods, but especially flaxseed, soy and alfalfa. By reducing their level of male hormones and increasing their female hormones, we can prevent their shape from becoming too masculine, and also stimulate weight loss from the abdomen and trunk. Android women often crave high GI carbohydrates, which will increase insulin levels and lead to abdominal obesity. They need to choose low GI carbohydrates such as legumes, raw nuts, seeds and whole grains. If they choose the unhealthy fats such as deep fried foods and hydrogenated vegetable oils in combination with too much refined sugar, they will often develop a fatty liver.

Android women benefit from nutrients that can:-

- Balance their hormones so that excess levels of male hormones (androgens) are reduced and the levels of female hormones (oestrogen and progesterone) are maintained. This will make the figure line more feminine and increase weight loss from the abdomen and trunk. This will also help to reduce the signs of excessive male hormones such as acne, facial and body hair, and scalp hair loss.
  Hops is probably the most oestrogenic of all the herbs and its female effect can be augmented with Red Clover and Dong Quai.
- Improve their liver function so that the ability of the liver to burn fat increases. This will reduce abdominal obesity and restore the waistline. Other benefits of improved liver function are lowered cholesterol levels and improvement of blood sugar metabolism. Syndrome X can be controlled and usually

reversed completely, with improved liver function and weight loss. St. Mary's Thistle, Choline and Inositol are beneficial lipotrophic factors for the liver. The term lipotrophic means beneficial for the function of the liver.

- Android women can benefit from natural fibre such as chitosan, which reduces the absorption of saturated fat from the foods in the diet. This will reduce the amount of fat returning back to the liver from the gut after eating. Chitosan is a proven substance for reducing the absorption of fat.

Weight control nutrients for Android Body Type

Chitosan 250 mg
St. Mary's Thistle 25mg
Red Clover 25mg
Hops 25 mg
Dong Quai 25 mg
Choline 12.5mg
Inositol 12.5mg
Take 3 times daily before food

Gynaeoid Body Type

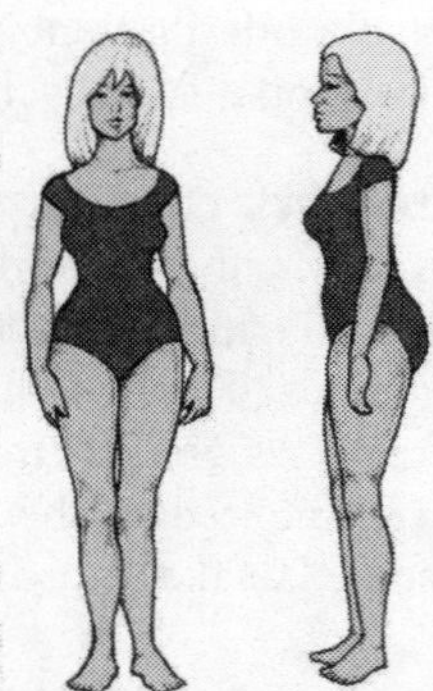

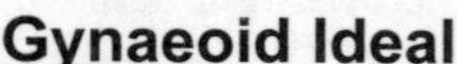

Gynaeoid Ideal

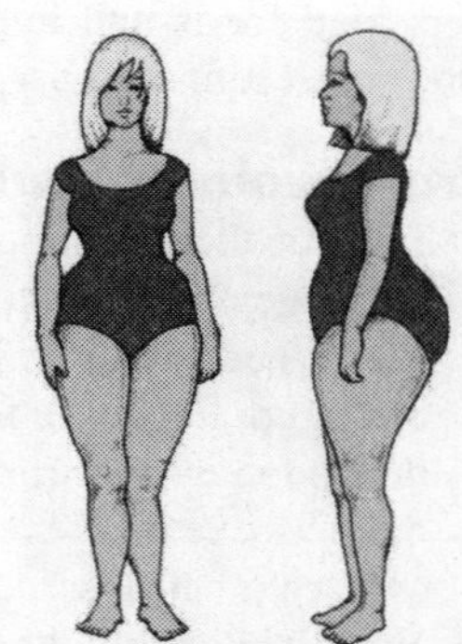

Gynaeoid Overweight

Approximately 40% of women belong to this body type, which is characterised by small to medium shoulders, a narrow tapering waistline and wide hips. Weight gain tends to occur on the buttocks and thighs, which further accentuates the pear shape of the Gynaeoid type. The hips and thighs curve outwards and weight gain occurs only below the waistline. Gynaeoid women are "oestrogen dominant", which means that the hormone oestrogen has the greatest influence in their body shape. They often have a relative deficiency of the other female hormone called progesterone. Excessive oestrogen promotes fat deposition and cellulite around the hips, thighs and buttocks. Progesterone balances the effect of oestrogen and helps to reduce weight from the hips and thighs.

The Gynaeoid body type is uncommon in men, however very occasionally you will find a man who falls into this category.

Gynaeoid women tend to crave foods that combine fat and refined sugars such as chocolate, custards, gooey creamy cakes, cream biscuits, and ice cream. These food combinations increase their sensitivity to the female hormone oestrogen, which will further accentuate weight gain around the buttocks and thighs. Gynaeoid women should avoid these high-fat high-sugar food combinations, and eat natural sugars from fruit, fruit sorbets and dried fruits.

Gynaeoid women benefit from nutrients that can:-

- Increase natural progesterone production in the body
- Reduce oestrogen dominance
- Reduce cravings for sweet creamy foods
- Reduce cellulite in the buttocks and thighs
- Reduce fluid retention in the buttocks and thighs

These actions will reduce the fat building effect of oestrogen on the buttocks and thighs, enabling weight loss from these areas. Fat will be more readily metabolised and converted into muscle.

Weight loss will occur from the buttocks and thighs, and not from the face and breasts.

Gynaeoid women often lack progesterone and the use of natural progesterone can facilitate weight loss from the buttocks and thighs, thus reducing their pear shape.

Weight control nutrients for Gynaeoid Body Type

Wild Yam 150 mg
Parsley Piert 25 mg
Vitex Agnes Castus 50mg
Gymnema Sylvestre 25mg
Chromium picolinate 67 mcg
Take 3 times daily before food

Thyroid Body Type

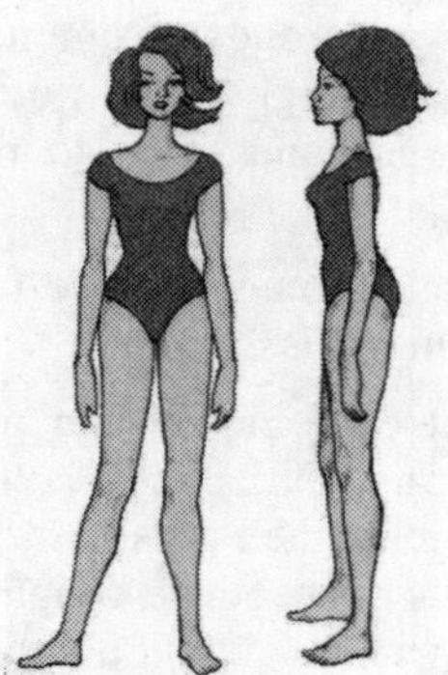

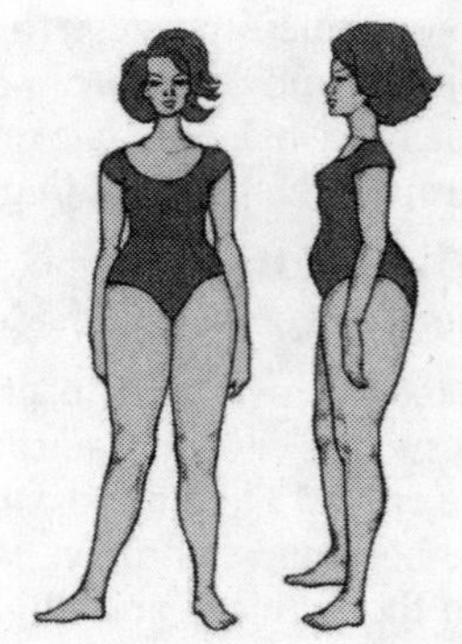

Thyroid Ideal **Thyroid Overweight**

Approximately 10% of women and 5% of men belong to this body type, which is characterised by a fine (small) bone structure, relatively long limbs compared to the trunk and a long narrow neck. Thyroid shaped people often become dancers or fashion models, and can be described as having a 'race-horse' or 'grey-hound' appearance.

Thyroid types have a high metabolic rate and do not gain weight easily, so that they can often eat much larger amounts than their friends without showing the effects. We call them thyroid types because they have such a rapid and efficient metabolism, and not because they are more likely to suffer with thyroid diseases.

Interestingly thyroid women are often naughty with their diet, in that they miss meals and live on stimulants, such as caffeine, diet sodas, fizzy soft drinks, sugar and cigarettes.

Blood sugar imbalances often result from the overuse of stimulants, which may lead to fatigue, but Thyroid types try to overcome this with more stimulants!

Caffeine, nicotine, diet pills, artificial sweeteners etc, are often the "more the better" for Thyroid types, who consume stimulants in excess, with few side effects until chronic "burn out" supervenes.

They are more likely to suffer with anorexia nervosa than are other body types, or may suffer with less severe eating disorders, which can cause their weight to fluctuate dramatically. Overall they do not put on weight easily, and if they become very underweight, especially in combination with smoking and a deficiency of nutrients, their oestrogen levels may become very low. Low oestrogen levels lead to a reversible loss of breast tissue and feminine curves, absence or irregularity of menstrual bleeding, and in the long term poor spinal posture and osteoporosis. I encourage thyroid types to eat small frequent meals containing protein and complex carbohydrates in the form of eggs, seafood, poultry, whole-grains, nuts, seeds and legumes. This will stabilise their metabolism and blood sugar levels, which will have a calming and balancing effect upon their nervous system.

Thyroid women benefit from nutrients that can: -

- Improve the function of their adrenal glands thus producing increased and sustained energy levels.
- Reduce cravings for stimulants and sugary foods, which will make it much easier to follow a healthy eating program.
- Reduce the lows in blood sugar levels and energy, so typical of this body type.
- Increase the conversion of fat into muscle.
- Reduce stress levels.

Weight control nutrients for Thyroid Body Type

Chromium picolinate 67 mcg
Glutamine 100 mg
Liquorice 75 mg
Ginseng 75 mg
Magnesium chelate 200 mg
Zinc chelate 2 mg
Vitamin B 5, 10 mg
Take 3 times daily before food

Lymphatic Body Type

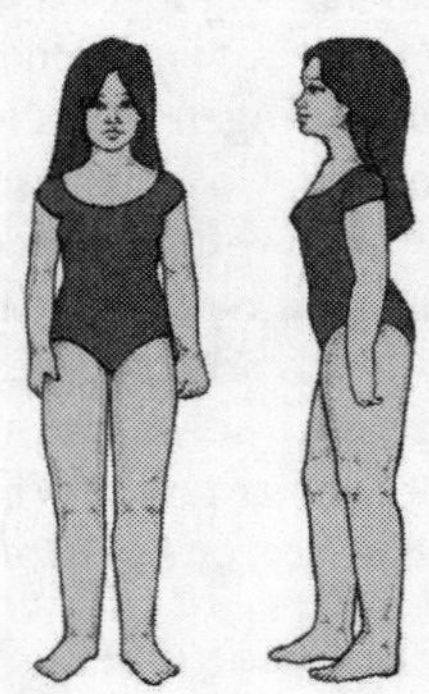

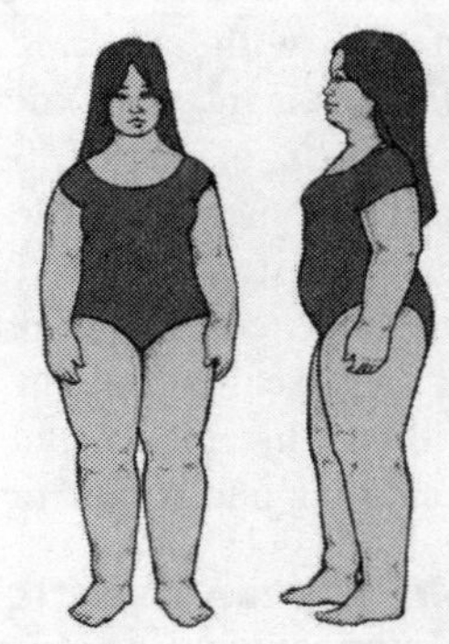

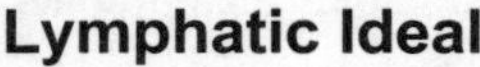

Lymphatic Ideal **Lymphatic Overweight**

Approximately 10% of women and 5% of men belong to this body type, which is characterised by weight gain all over the body.

The limbs have a thick puffy appearance and the bone structure is not very visible. It is as if there is a layer of fat all over the body, which is excessively thick. These people have often been plagued with weight excess since childhood. Lymphatic people have a very slow metabolic rate, which causes them to gain weight very easily. They also have an inefficient lymphatic system, which leads to fluid retention and makes lymphatic people appear fatter than they really are. Cellulite is common in this body type, with deposits of fat swollen with lymphatic fluid, giving a dimpled appearance on thick puffy limbs.

Lymphatic types may have imbalances in pituitary hormones, such as prolactin and growth hormone mediators, and overall they are hypersensitive to hormones. Lymphatic people tend to crave high fat dairy products such as full cream milk, butter, cheese, cream, ice cream and chocolate. Dairy products will overload their lymphatic system, and cause weight gain and fluid retention. I have found that lymphatic people should avoid all dairy products, and indeed if they follow a "liver cleansing diet" they can often lose weight quite easily for the first time in their lives. In lymphatic types, it is what you eat, rather than how much you eat that is important in speeding up metabolism and weight loss. An under active thyroid gland is more common in lymphatic types, so it is important that they keep a regular check on their thyroid function.

Lymphatic women benefit from nutrients that can:-

- Boost their sluggish metabolic rate
- Relieve fluid retention
- Eliminate mucus and toxins
- Improve the lymphatic system

Weight control nutrients for Lymphatic Body Type

Fenugreek 200mg
Rutin 50mg
Selenomethionine 4mcg
Celery 12.5mg
Horseradish 12.5mg
Fennel 12.5mg
Kelp 25mg
Cayenne fruit powder 2.5mg
Vitamin B 6, 2.5mg
Take 3 times daily before food

The Apple Shape versus the Pear Shape

Apple shaped people accumulate excess weight in the trunk and the abdomen.

Apple shaped women who carry most of their body fat around the abdomen may be at an increased risk of diabetes after the menopause. This also applies to men as they get older. These people are commonly Android or Lymphatic Body Types and are more resistant to insulin than those who store most of their body fat in the hips and thighs. The latter are known as pear shaped or Gynaeoid Body Types. According to Dr Cynthia Sites from the University of Vermont College of Medicine in Burlington, "efforts to reduce either subcutaneous abdominal fat or intra-abdominal fat should be helpful in reducing the risk of type 2 diabetes in post menopausal women". Their study measured abdominal fat and total body fat and determined its relationship to insulin sensitivity. They found that the higher the abdominal fat stores were, the less the body was able to respond to insulin. It is well known that higher levels of body fat are associated with a higher risk of type 2 diabetes, however the effect of body fat distribution upon insulin resistance in peri-menopausal women had not been fully explored. The results published in the January 2001 issue of The Journal of Fertility and Sterility, showed that women with lower amounts of abdominal fat were less likely to develop Syndrome X and diabetes, than women with higher amounts of abdominal fat.

The apple shape is a common body shape, especially in men, but is also common in women.

How do you know if you are apple shaped?

- **Measure** your waist and hips with a tape measure while unclothed. To do this measure your waist an inch above the navel, or at its narrowest part, while standing with the abdominal muscles relaxed. If there is no smallest area around the waist, take the measurement at the level of the navel. Then measure your hips at their widest point while standing.
- **Divide** your waist measurement by your hip measurement to get your waist to hip ratio.

A waist to hip ratio of over 0.8 for women, and over 1.0 for men is suggestive of an unfavourable accumulation of fat around the middle, which occurs in apple shaped persons.

What causes excess fat deposits in the middle?

Hereditary factors
Alcohol excess
Smoking
Stress
Lack of exercise
Excess intake of unhealthy fats
Excess intake of refined carbohydrates and sugar
Excess intake or body production of male hormones
Syndrome X

Why is excess abdominal fat dangerous?

Fat cells in the abdominal area release fats into the blood stream more easily than fat cells located in other areas of the body. Release of fat from abdominal fat cells begins 3 to 4 hours after eating, compared to many more hours after eating for fat cells located elsewhere in the body. The early release of fat produces higher levels of triglycerides and free fatty acids in the blood stream. This increases insulin resistance. Abdominal fat cells release their fatty acids straight to the liver, which increases the risk of fatty liver and metabolic problems.

The risk of heart disease goes up two and a half times for men with diabetes and the apple shaped physique, and rises eightfold for women with diabetes and the apple shape.

Hormonal case history

Rona came to see me complaining of abdominal weight gain, abdominal bloating, fatigue and facial hair. She was an apple shaped woman with all her weight excess in the trunk and abdomen, and had a large "liver roll" around her upper abdomen. Clinical assessment revealed that she had all the chemical imbalances of Syndrome X, with high triglycerides, low HDL cholesterol, and raised fasting insulin levels. An ultrasound scan of her upper abdomen revealed that she had a fatty liver. Her liver enzymes were slightly elevated, consistent with liver inflammation from fatty infiltration. She weighed 95 kilograms and although she was quite tall, she looked very overweight. She had widespread facial hair, which she controlled with regular waxing. Blood tests revealed excess levels of male hormones with an elevated free androgen index.

Rona had undergone a total hysterectomy with removal of both ovaries 10 years previously. Thus not surprisingly, her levels of the female hormones oestrogen and progesterone were non-existent. Rona needed natural oestrogen and progesterone replacement therapy to balance her hormones, which would reduce her excessive male hormones. I prescribed these hormones in the form of a cream, which she rubbed into the inside skin of her upper arm twice daily. In her case I preferred the use of hormone creams instead of tablets or lozenges, as I did not want to over work her fatty liver. Rona was started on a supplement to reduce insulin resistance, and a liver tonic powder, and instructed to follow the Syndrome X eating plan.

Rona was accustomed to eating a lot of carbohydrates, and her diet was deficient in raw foods, essential fatty acids and protein. She did not find the change in her way of eating difficult, as once her insulin levels started to come down, she no longer felt so hungry and lost her cravings for sugary foods. Her energy levels improved as her insulin and blood sugar levels came down into the normal range.

Six months after beginning her program Rona had lost 25 kilograms, with all the weight loss due to the reduction in excess fat from her trunk and abdomen. Her bloating had gone and she was able to wear belts and jeans again. Blood tests revealed normal levels of her male hormones, which was very desirable as this had reduced her facial hair and insulin resistance. Her excessive levels of male hormones had been coming from the fat in her upper body, and her adrenal glands, and these male hormones had been increasing her insulin resistance and weight-gaining tendency.

This case history shows how important it is to balance not only the insulin levels, but also any imbalances, which exist in other body hormones such as the sex hormones and thyroid hormones.

16

Chapter Sixteen

Hormonal Imbalances and weight gain

Hormonal Imbalances and weight gain

Are hormonal imbalances making you fat?

Years ago doctors, family members and friends would often advise women who battled with a weight problem that it was due to "hormonal problems" or their "glands". In those days there was very little understanding about the ways that hormones affected the body. No real help was available and the patient just accepted that this was the way she/he had to remain. Today things have improved greatly and we now know that specific hormones can affect metabolism, and also the areas where excessive fat will be deposited. We are able to measure accurately the blood levels of all the body's hormones, and can pin point the significant hormonal imbalances that will trigger weight gain.

Thyroid Gland Dysfunction

Dysfunction of the thyroid gland can have a profound effect on the metabolism. An overactive thyroid gland produces excess amounts of thyroid hormone, which results in weight loss even though there is a voracious appetite. Conversely, an under active thyroid gland does not produce adequate amounts of thyroid hormone and the metabolism slows down. The symptoms of thyroid gland underactivity are weight gain, fluid retention, bloating, low body temperature, constipation, hair loss, dryness of the skin and a general slowing of bodily and mental functions. The condition of thyroid gland underactivity is called Hypothyroidism, while the condition of an over active thyroid gland is called Hyperthyroidism.

Hypothyroidism is very common in middle aged persons, especially peri-menopausal women. It is associated with fatigue and muscle weakness, so there is not much inclination to exercise, which leads to more weight gain.

The function of the thyroid gland can be easily checked with a simple blood test, which measures the level of the thyroid hormones. The thyroid gland produces the hormone called thyroxine, which is also known as T4. Thyroxine (T4) must be converted in the body into the active form of thyroid hormone, which is known as triiodothyronine or T3. The active form of thyroid hormone (T3) directly stimulates the energy factories inside the cells to burn food calories at a faster rate. This is why those with an over-active thyroid gland lose weight, even though they are eating much more than normal.

The blood tests for thyroid gland function must measure at least the following three hormones –

HORMONE	NORMAL RANGE
Thyroid Stimulating Hormone (TSH)	(0.5 to 5.0) mIU/L
Free T 4	(9.0 to 24.0) pmol/L
Free T 3	(2.2 to 5.4) pmol/L

If the T 4 and/or T 3 levels are found to be below the normal ranges, and the TSH is found to be above the normal range, we can say that the thyroid gland is under active.

If the thyroid gland is only slightly under active, we are often able to stimulate it back to normal function by the following –

Improving the diet and lifestyle

Taking supplemental magnesium tablets

Taking supplemental selenium 100 to 200mcg daily

Taking a mixture of the trace minerals manganese, zinc, iodine (often in the form of kelp) and chromium

Taking supplemental flaxseed oil and evening primrose oil

Taking supplemental Vitamin E

If however the thyroid function remains abnormally low after 3 months of nutritional supplementation, it will be necessary to take thyroid hormone replacement. This is usually given in the form of tablets containing thyroxine hormone. Many people worry that taking thyroxine tablets is the same as taking artificial drugs, however this is not correct, as thyroxine tablets are merely replacing a natural hormone that the thyroid gland can no longer produce by itself. If the dosage is carefully controlled, there are generally no side effects.

In most people the thyroxine tablets work very well and increase the metabolic rate back to normal, so that weight loss begins and energy levels are restored.

In some people the thyroxine tablets have a good initial response, but become increasingly ineffective over time. This condition is called "**thyroid resistance**", and means that the body cells have become resistant to the effect of the hormone thyroxine (T4). This can be compared to Syndrome X, where the body cells have become resistant to the effects of the hormone insulin.

In those with **thyroid resistance**, the body is not able to convert the thyroxine (T4) into its active form of triiodothyronine (T3), so the metabolism slows down. To treat thyroid resistance we can use supplemental selenium and essential fatty acids to help the conversion of T4 into T3. This will work in some cases of thyroid resistance, however in very resistant cases it will be necessary to give triiodothyronine (T3) tablets. T3 tablets are known as Tertroxin tablets. Generally speaking in cases of severe thyroid resistance we need to give both Thyroxine (T4) and Tertroxin (T3) tablets, to restore normal thyroid hormone balance and metabolism. Typical doses are Thyroxine 100 to 150mcg and Tertroxin 10mcg twice daily. You will need a prescription for these medications and will need to be monitored by your doctor.

In people with **thyroid resistance**, the addition of Tertroxin (T3) tablets can be dramatically effective and enable the patient to lose weight much more easily. I have also found that by treating thyroid problems correctly we are able to improve Syndrome X, as thyroid hormones are so vitally important in controlling cholesterol levels and metabolism. If you have Syndrome X and are finding that you cannot lose weight, and feel fatigued, I recommend that you ask your doctor to fully evaluate your thyroid gland function. Sluggish thyroid function could be the hidden problem that is preventing you from being successful with your weight loss program.

Adrenal Gland Dysfunction

Adrenal hormones

The hormone cortisol is made in the adrenal glands, and is important in regulating metabolism and the immune system. Excessive levels of cortisol can cause a moon shaped face, fluid retention, bloating and weight gain around the neck, trunk and abdomen.

If stress levels are very high or prolonged, the adrenal glands may pump out excessive cortisol, and this is why severe stress can lead to weight gain in some people. If stress is preventing you from losing weight, I suggest that you take some anti-stress nutrients such as magnesium, vitamin B complex and vitamin C, along with the herb hypericum.

Just as the seasons come and go in a predictable manner, so do our hormonal cycles. The adrenal glands have a circadian or diurnal rhythm, and release higher amounts of cortisol, adrenalin and androgens in the early hours of the morning. This hormonal surge is needed to help us awake and face the challenges of the new day. By sunset the levels of these hormones are significantly lower, which allows us to relax and gradually unwind for restful sleep. Prolonged stress can cause chronic elevation of the stress hormone adrenalin, which will raise the blood sugar level, thus aggravating insulin resistance. In some people this can lead to weight gain.

Menopause and Weight Gain

Hormonal imbalances are very common during menopause

- The post war baby boomers are arriving at menopause in unprecedented numbers, and the average human life span has increased dramatically in the last century. In today's society, is it really a natural thing for a woman to spend over one third of her life without sex hormones in her body? Women now rightfully have greater expectations of their older years, and they wish to avoid osteoporosis, heart disease, obesity and mental decline. We now have the knowledge to prevent these things that used to be considered a normal part of ageing.

- Artificial chemicals, which resemble oestrogen (known as xeno-estrogens) are present in our environment from pesticides, insecticides, solvents and plastics. These xeno-estrogens can damage the ovaries, leading to hormonal imbalances such as infertility and premature menopause. It is only the liver that can break down these toxic chemicals so that they can be eliminated from the body. It is always important to improve the liver function in cases of hormonal imbalances.

- Anabolic steroids may be used in the production of meat and poultry for human consumption. These strong hormones may cause weight gain, and hormonal imbalances in menopausal women. Choosing organically raised produce can help these problems.

How do hormones get into our body?

- **From our diet** – plant foods contain phyto-sterols, which have a balancing effect upon our cell's sex hormone receptors. Animal sourced foods such as land-based meats (red meat, pork, and chicken) and dairy products, contain animal hormones, which have a more masculine effect upon our cell receptors. We need to increase the consumption of plant based foods in our diet such as legumes (beans, peas and lentils), nuts, seeds, unprocessed grains, fruits and vegetables.
- Most people know that our hormones are **manufactured in our various glands**, such as the thyroid gland, the adrenal glands, the ovaries and testicles. However it may come as a surprise to you to learn that hormones are also **manufactured in our fatty tissues**. Excessive amounts of upper level body fat produce more male hormones (androgens), which can increase insulin resistance and the risk of Syndrome X. Excessive production of androgens may cause "androgenisation", resulting in facial and body hair, acne, thinning of the hair in a male pattern, and menstrual irregularity. This is what we find in many women with polycystic ovarian syndrome, especially if they carry a lot of weight in the upper body and abdomen.
  Lower body fat produces female hormones, such as the weak oestrogen called oestrone, which if excessive can increase fat deposits and cellulite in the thighs and buttocks.
- **Hormones are prescribed** in the form of the oral contraceptive pill, which contains synthetic hormones and hormone replacement therapy (HRT) for menopause. HRT is used in both men and women to replace the sex hormones that they are no longer able to produce in adequate amounts. There are many different types of HRT, ranging from weaker natural hormones to more potent synthetic hormones. The type of HRT or oral contraceptive chosen can have a big influence upon your metabolism and your weight gain.

What can we do about hormonal imbalances?

- Balance our diet – eat more plant-based foods, and use herbal formulas containing combinations of Black Cohosh, Dong Quai, Sarsaparilla, Sage, Liquorice root, Wild Yam, Kelp and Horsetail.

- Maintain a healthy body weight through a balanced diet and regular exercise programs.
- Use more feminine oral contraceptive pills such as Marvelon, Femoden and Diane. These contain the more "friendly" or neutral progestagens such as desogestrel and gestodene, which are less likely to cause weight gain than are the masculine progestagens, such as levo-norgestrel and norethisterone. The anti-male hormone called Androcur can reduce the effect of excessive male hormones, which will reduce insulin resistance. It is important to choose hormones for contraception, or hormone replacement therapy that are able to reduce the excess levels of male hormones that we find in some women. This will reduce their insulin resistance and make it much easier for them to lose weight. It is easy for your doctor to check your level of male hormones (androgens) with a simple blood test, which measures the total testosterone and free androgen index in your body. These tests are most worthwhile if you believe that your hormones could be sabotaging your efforts to lose weight.
- Use natural hormones such as progesterone cream or lozenges for premenstrual syndrome instead of synthetic hormones, which tend to cause weight gain.
- Use Hormone Replacement Therapy (HRT) that is more natural and does not overwork the liver. Hormone creams containing mixtures of natural hormones (such as oestradiol, progesterone, and DHEA), or hormone patches, will bypass the liver. These types of hormones are absorbed into the blood stream through the skin and do not pass directly through the liver. For this reason they are less likely to cause weight gain than hormone tablets. Every woman is an individual, and blood tests are required to determine tailor made HRT. In general by using lower doses of natural hormones that bypass the liver, we are able to avoid weight gain at menopause in women who are predisposed to obesity.
- **The Women's Health Advisory Service can help women to find doctors who are skilled in the technique of using natural hormones and phyto-estrogens to overcome hormonal imbalances. Call 02 4655 8855 for more information.**

Common questions about hormones and weight gain

What is the difference between natural and synthetic hormones?

Natural hormones are chemically identical to the hormones produced by your own glands, which means that your body cannot tell the difference between your own hormones and a natural hormone prescribed by your doctor. Natural hormones are made in the laboratory from plant hormones found in yams and soybeans, by making slight physical changes to the plant hormone's molecular structure. Natural hormones can be prescribed in the form of creams, lozenges, tablets, injections, patches, implants and pessaries.

Synthetic hormones have a different chemical structure to your body's own hormones, and are more difficult for the liver to breakdown (metabolise). This makes synthetic hormones stronger and more likely to cause side effects than natural hormones. Sometimes this increased potency can be desirable when we use strong synthetic hormones to overcome severe endometriosis or to reduce dangerously heavy menstrual bleeding. The hormones used in the oral contraceptive pill need to be synthetic because natural hormones are not strong enough to prevent ovulation from occurring. However where possible it is safer and better accepted by the patient to use natural hormones when we are treating problems such as premenstrual syndrome, post-natal depression, post tubal ligation problems and menopause. One of the main reasons for this is that the natural hormones are less likely to cause mood disorders and weight gain.

What are plant hormones and can they help me?

Plant foods such as legumes, nuts, seeds, whole-grains and some herbs, fruits and vegetables contain sex hormones, and we call these phyto-sterols. If they have an oestrogenic or female effect we call them "phyto-estrogens". We know that populations, who consume abundant and regular amounts of dietary phyto-estrogens, have a lower incidence of breast cancer and other hormone sensitive cancers. This is because phyto-estrogens have a balancing effect upon cellular hormone receptors, which means they can protect the cell against over-stimulation from sex hormones that are produced in the body. All women and indeed men as well, should regularly consume plenty of plant hormones from the above foods to promote hormonal balance, a healthy immune system and to reduce the risk of cancer. Herbs containing beneficial plant hormones are black cohosh, dong quai, liquorice, red clover, sage and hops. Foods that are high in beneficial plant hormones are soybeans and their products, flaxseeds (linseeds) and alfalfa. Supplements and/or foods containing phyto-estrogens can help with premenstrual syndrome, breast tenderness, endometriosis, heavy bleeding, menopausal symptoms and hair loss. You can obtain these herbs individually or combined, from a health food store or pharmacy.

For more information call the Health Advisory Service on 02 4655 8855.

Menopause

Most women begin the peri-menopause at some time during their 40s, which is really the beginning of ovarian failure. The peri-menopause consists of the period of time, before, during and after menopause, where the ovarian output of sex hormones becomes erratic and eventually fails completely. Menopause occurs because the ovaries run out of eggs (follicles), and the average age is 50 years, with an average range from 45 to 55 years.

A small percentage of women (around one in a hundred), have a premature menopause in their thirties or early forties, and rarely, I have seen women in their early twenties go through menopause. The causes of premature menopause vary from chronic stress, autoimmune diseases, smoking, genetic factors, hysterectomy, removal of the ovaries, chemotherapy and in some cases are unknown. Other women continue to produce good levels of oestrogen and progesterone right through their forties, and well into their fifties, before the ovaries eventually fail. No matter what age a woman goes through menopause, the question of whether to take hormone replacement therapy (HRT) remains an individual one.

The best way to assess the relative benefits of HRT is to look at the profile of a high-risk menopausal woman who would generally do better with HRT, and a low risk menopausal woman in whom HRT is optional.

Profile of a Low-Risk Menopausal Woman

Menopause at age 50, plus or minus 5 years
No family history of cardiovascular disease before the age of 65
No family history of osteoporosis
Good bone density as determined from a bone scan
Medium to heavy bone (skeletal) structure
No history of depression
A healthy nutrient rich diet
Non-smoker
Regular weight bearing exercise and aerobic exercise
No long term use of drugs that would increase bone loss (eg. steroids, high doses of thyroid medication, some diuretics)
A healthy cardiovascular system
Happy disposition and good relationships

Profile of a High-Risk Menopausal Woman

Premature menopause (age 40 or earlier)
Artificial menopause before the age of 45, caused by surgery, drugs, radiation or chemotherapy
Cardiovascular disease
Strong family history of cardiovascular disease
Strong family history of Alzheimer's dementia
Sedentary life-style
Poor nutrient deficient diet
Sexual dysfunction and poor relationships
Depression and lack of enjoyment in life
Smoking
Fine bone structure
Low bone density as determined from a bone scan

Hormone Replacement Therapy

The art and science of hormone replacement therapy (HRT) has blossomed in the last 5 years, because we can now tailor make combinations of natural hormones to suit every individual woman.

During the first few years of menopause, prescriptions for HRT must be continually fine-tuned with regular adjustments in the doses of the various hormones. This is because a woman's body, life expectations, symptoms and sexuality is continually evolving as she ages. The goal of natural HRT is to restore hormones to around the normal body levels that were present during a woman's thirties or forties. An integrative or holistic approach, balancing all three classes of body hormones (oestrogen, progesterone, and androgen) is ideal, even in women who have had a hysterectomy. Currently most women who have had a hysterectomy are offered only oestrogens, without consideration of the need for progesterone or androgens. Many different combinations of hormones, including oestrogens, progesterone, testosterone, and DHEA, can be administered in different ways, such as patches, tablets, injections, creams, implants and lozenges (troches). Because there are so many choices I recommend beginning with a blood test to evaluate your own hormonal profile before starting any HRT.

There are three types of oestrogen that are produced in the female body. These are oestrone (E1), oestradiol (E2), and oestriol (E3). Oestrone is produced in significant amounts in lower level body fat, which is one reason that bigger women often have a later menopause, have less osteoporosis and do not have such severe symptoms of menopause, such as hot flushes and vaginal dryness. Conversely, women who are underweight with low body fat will often have more severe menopausal symptoms and require higher doses of HRT. The most commonly prescribed forms of HRT are oestradiol and oestrone, which are available in a wide variety of forms. The weakest of all the body oestrogens is oestriol, which makes it a good choice for women with any risk factors for breast cancer or those with only mild symptoms.

The main advantages of oestrogen replacement therapy are that it elevates the good cholesterol (HDL), and promotes healthy blood vessel walls, and this is why oestrogen replacement has been linked with a reduced risk of cardiovascular disease. Oestrogen also reduces the rate of bone loss, although by itself it will not build bone. Progesterone and testosterone are also beneficial for bone density.

No matter what age you go through menopause, you will have fewer symptoms and feel healthier if you have a good diet, a regular exercise program, a positive state of mind and a healthy liver and adrenal glands. The liver breaks down (metabolises) all the body's hormones, as well as any HRT that is being prescribed. If the liver is sluggish or dysfunctional, hormonal imbalances can arise. Peri-menopausal women with sluggish liver function are more likely to have a weight problem, because the liver is the major fat burning organ in the body. The adrenal glands are very important during the peri-menopausal years because they take over the role of the failed ovaries to a significant degree, and continue to produce significant amounts of the sex hormones, including androgens. Women with healthy adrenal glands have much better energy levels and sex drive.

Women in their fifties and sixties will often want to continue with some form of nutritional and/or hormonal support for the post-menopausal years, with the aim of reducing osteoporosis and cardiovascular disease. During these two decades the body produces less and less sex hormones and this can cause continuing bone loss, increased cholesterol levels and sexual dysfunction. In these age groups lower doses of oestrogen replacement are required, and this is ideally given in the form of patches, creams or troches. If older women are troubled by sexual and/or bladder dysfunction, troches and/or creams combining small doses of oestrogen along with testosterone, and if needed progesterone, work extremely well.

The major health problems for women over 50 are osteoporosis, a higher risk of cancer and cardiovascular diseases. Weight excess is also more common in these age groups and is commonly associated with Syndrome X and/or thyroid gland dysfunction.

It is important that women utilise preventative strategies to reduce the occurrence of these common diseases. To keep these diseases in check some simple yet powerful dietary strategies can be followed such as —

- Drinking at least 8 glasses of filtered water daily
- Buy a juice-extracting machine and drink fresh juices made from raw vegetables to increase your intake of anti-oxidants and improve liver function.
- Buy an inexpensive coffee grinder or food processor to grind fresh raw nuts and seeds such as flaxseeds, sesame seeds, sunflower seeds, almonds and pumpkin seeds etc. to provide essential fatty acids, phyto-estrogens and minerals
- Diversify your sources of protein from seafood, eggs, free range chicken, lean red fresh meats, legumes, whole-grains, nuts, seeds and protein powder. Ensure that you eat regular protein at least three times daily, as this will help you control your weight and reduce sugar cravings. It is also essential for those with the common metabolic disturbance of Syndrome X.
- Use super foods which are nutrient dense, to support the skeleton and blood vessels such as brewers yeast, spirulina, fresh wheat germ, garlic, onions, citrus fruits, kelp, wheat grass, alfalfa, beans, fresh sprouts, cold pressed oils, tahini, hummus, avocados, lecithin and apple cider vinegar.
- Do a regular exercise program including walking, swimming, recreational sports, lightweights, yoga or tai chi.

In all peri-menopausal and post-menopausal women, even those on HRT, nutritional supplements can be of great help in reducing osteoporosis and cardiovascular disease, and help to slow down the ageing process.

The most useful supplements can be combined into what I call a "Natural Menopause Kit".

- Essential fatty acids - from evening primrose oil, flaxseed oil, lecithin (available in one capsule), and ground seeds and nuts and oily fish, such as sardines, salmon and tuna.
- Minerals - selenium, calcium hydroxyapatite, zinc, manganese, silica, and magnesium to protect the skeleton
- Vitamins - E, D, K and C to maintain bone density and healthy immune function.
- Phyto-estrogenic herbs and foods
- Organic sulphur such as MSM can help to reduce the symptoms of menopause and reduce hair loss and ageing of the skin.

Phyto-estrogen Table

ISOFLAVONES – genistein, diadzein, biochanin A, formononetin

Found in -

Legumes-chickpeas, lentils, beans especially soybeans and alfalfa sprouts
Some vegetables
Some herbs - liquorice, sage, hops, clovers
Alcoholic drinks

LIGNANS

Lignans are converted to substances with biological oestrogenic effects in the body

Found in -

Seeds and nuts, eg. linseed (flaxseed), sesame, sunflower, pumpkin seeds, seed oils, and whole legumes
Fruits and vegetables
Whole grains and dried seaweeds

COUMESTANS

Coumestrol is the collective name for the 20 coumestans that have been identified, and is the most potent of the phyto-estrogens. It may be 30-100 times more active as an oestrogen than isoflavones, although theoretically 200 times less potent then oestrone.

Coumestrol Containing plants –

Soybean sprouts, alfalfa sprouts, soybeans dry, green string beans,
Green and red beans, mung beans, split peas and red clover

HEALTH BENEFITS OF ISOFLAVONES & LIGNANS

- Anti-oxidants
- Reduction of osteoporosis
- Reduction of heart disease
- Reduction of menopausal symptoms
- Cancer preventative

Plants containing phyto-estrogens are on the list of cancer preventative foods that have been studied within the USA Designer Food Program – this includes liquorice, soybeans, linseed, barley, the Brassicaceae (cabbage) and Umbelliferae (celery) families

The ingestion of plants in the Brassicaceae family is strongly associated with a reduction in breast, colon, lung and other cancers.

Premenstrual Syndrome and Weight Gain

The pre-menopausal ovaries have a cycle, which approximates 28 days, and is controlled by the development and release of a follicle (egg) from the ovary. Typically the egg is released from the ovary on day 14 of this cycle, and this is called ovulation. During the 2 weeks before ovulation, the ovaries produce increasing amounts of oestrogen, which peaks in the 2 to 3 days before ovulation. Oestrogen is an up-beat hormone promoting energy, creativity and libido, so that you will feel very perky on these high oestrogen days. Immediately after ovulation occurs your oestrogen levels take a temporary dive for several days, which may make you less outgoing and a little moody. Immediately after ovulation the ovary starts to manufacture progesterone, which tones down your up-beat oestrogen and makes the next 10 days pass at a slower pace. Progesterone will make you feel more relaxed and self-contented, so that this is a good time to meditate, think things through and pamper yourself.

The most testing zone of the monthly menstrual cycle is the 4 days before menstrual bleeding commences, because both oestrogen and progesterone levels are dropping to very low levels. This may cause unpleasant symptoms of the pre-menstrual syndrome, and is a time where your body and mind are more sensitive to all forms of stress. Try to get extra rest, drink plenty of fluids, and avoid alcohol and too many excesses at this time. This vulnerable and tense zone is relieved by the onset of the menstrual bleeding, which causes a sense of physical and mental release once bleeding becomes established. During the premenstrual phase of the cycle, the drop in sex hormones may cause excess fluctuations in blood sugar levels and fluid retention. Some women get very strong cravings for carbohydrates and sugar during this phase and can easily put on several kilograms of weight. To avoid premenstrual weight gain and fluid retention, you need to follow the eating plan in this book very closely during this phase of the cycle. By eating regular first class protein and plenty of raw vegetables and fruits, you will find it much easier to prevent premenstrual weight gain. Taking a good liver tonic and extra essential fatty acids can also help to prevent these problems.

Weight gain after childbirth

I have met many women who have complained of large increases in their weight during and after pregnancy. Breast feeding your baby can help to keep your weight down, but in many women this is not enough to control their ballooning weight after childbirth.

The reasons for excessive weight gain during pregnancy and after childbirth include the following –

- The huge levels of hormones produced during pregnancy can increase the workload of the kidneys and liver, leading to fluid retention and an increased tendency to store fat. Women with a tendency to insulin resistance may find that they develop temporary diabetes of pregnancy, which is known as gestational diabetes. This worsening of insulin resistance often leads to a fat storing tendency.
- After the baby is born there is less personal time for exercise and sleep. Fatigue may result in less attention to meal preparation, making it easy to grab quick high carbohydrate snacks to keep energy levels up.
- Depression due to hormonal and life style changes may take away the motivation to follow a healthy eating plan and exercise program.

It is important to be aware of these risk factors and have a preventative plan to follow. Keep your liver and kidneys healthy by drinking plenty of water and raw vegetable juices. Have handy snacks available containing raw nuts, seeds and fruit, so you don't lose control and reach for the high sugar pick me ups. Keep the refrigerator stocked with plenty of high protein foods, such as cold roast beef and lamb, seafood (canned varieties of crabmeat, sardines, salmon and tuna are excellent), and eggs. Boiled eggs are a complete food, providing all essential amino acids. You can also use convenient cans of beans and combine them with nuts and seeds, or use a protein powder to obtain first class protein quickly. Remember that protein depletion can lead to muscle loss and increase cravings for high GI carbohydrates. Supplemental magnesium is very helpful for those with fluid retention and insulin resistance during pregnancy. Take a good liver tonic powder or capsules to keep your liver burning fat efficiently, and to help it cope with the high levels of hormones. If depression is a factor in causing you to eat badly, you may need to talk to your doctor about using a mild anti-depressant medication for 6 to 12 months. The effective treatment of depression can help with weight loss. In some women with post-natal depression and weight gain, the use of natural progesterone cream or lozenges can help greatly. Natural progesterone is also generally safe to take while breast-feeding.

It is important to act quickly if you find your self gaining large amounts of weight after childbirth, as I have seen many women put on huge amounts of weight in a short period of time. It is then much harder to lose the weight, especially if you do nothing about it for several years.

RESOURCES FOR WOMEN WITH HORMONAL PROBLEMS

Your family doctor is the best initial point of contact and you can be referred to a specialist gynaecologist or endocrinologist if needed.

The Hormonal Advisory Service: This service provides information/referral for natural hormone therapy, phyto-estrogens, post-natal depression, pre-menstrual syndrome and menopause. Phone number: 02 4655 8855

Books

Boost Your Energy, by Dr Sandra Cabot, discusses natural hormone therapy
Don't Let Hormones Ruin Your Life, by Dr Sandra Cabot
Natural Progesterone - the World's best kept Secret, by Jenny Birdsey
Menopause – HRT and its Natural Alternatives, by Dr Sandra Cabot
What your doctor does not tell you about menopause, Dr John Lee
The Menopause Industry, Sandra Coney
Osteoporosis - the silent epidemic, Dr Leonard Rose

Julie's Case History

Julie provides an interesting insight into the effect that the foods we eat everyday can have upon our hormones and weight. Julie was 40 years of age and had all the symptoms of polycystic ovarian syndrome with excess body hair, scalp hair loss, absent menstruation and a BMI of 31. She was addicted to bread and sweet pastries and found it very hard to control her weight. Julie decided to go on a high-protein high-fat diet consisting largely of ham and cheese. She did manage to lose a significant amount of weight on this diet, but found that she became generally unwell while eating large amounts of these high-protein high-fat foods. She found that she suffered with infections in the skin and sinuses and also noticed that her scalp hair began to fall out at a faster rate. Julie found that it was impossible to sustain this high-protein high-fat diet because of her poor health and increased hair loss.

To help Julie we came up with a high-protein low-fat diet, which did contain approximately 30% carbohydrate from low GI foods. I gave her recipes that provided first class protein from combining legumes, nuts and seeds as well as seafood and eggs. She was told to eat 2 salads and plenty of cooked vegetable everyday, and to avoid all breads and pastries. Although her weight loss was slower at first than it had been with the high-protein high-fat diet, she started to feel much better generally and found that her infections and hair loss stopped. In Julie's case the type of protein foods that she could tolerate were not dairy products and fatty meats, as these foods caused problems with her immune system and hormones. It was far better for her to choose more proteins from the plant food group and seafood, as these did not elevate her male hormone levels or overload her liver and immune system. Furthermore she had to have a diet that provided her with some carbohydrate, as otherwise she could not maintain a very restricted diet of only high-protein and high-fat foods. Provided she chose carbohydrates that were low GI and also provided her with first class protein, Julie would be able to control the chemical imbalance of Syndrome X, which was otherwise going to lead to severe obesity in her case. The types of protein foods and fats that you choose will have a profound effect upon your hormones and body shape, and will determine your long-term success.

Maggie's Case History

Maggie was typical of many women who come to see me trying to restore balance in their lives. For many women, physical and emotional balance can be elusive, especially since we cannot achieve one without the other. Maggie was 44 years old and had gained 20 kilograms since she went through menopause 2 years ago. She was an apple shaped woman, carrying all her excessive weight in the abdominal area and had a roll of fat around her upper abdomen.

She forced herself to avoid eating, but even when she did this, she did not lose weight. Maggie just kept on gaining weight and had become extremely frustrated. Her doctor had given her high doses of the hormone oestrogen in the form of Premarin tablets. These contain potent horse estrogens as well as human estrogens. Maggie did not realise that she had a fatty liver, and her poor dysfunctional liver could not cope with the strong hormones she was taking. Understandably they had caused more weight gain, and Maggie was trapped in a vicious cycle of ever increasing weight.

After testing Maggie, I confirmed that she had a fatty liver, slightly high cholesterol and elevated fasting insulin and blood sugar levels. She also felt hungry most of the time. Maggie was relieved to discover that she had a specific cause for her rapid weight gain - namely fatty liver and Syndrome X.

I stopped her Premarin tablets, and gave her a natural hormone cream containing natural human oestrogen and progesterone. This would be much better for her overworked liver, which could now get on with its job of burning fat. Maggie loved protein and vegetables, so the Syndrome X eating plan was easy for her to follow. She found that avoiding high GI carbohydrates, such as chips and processed breads, easily controlled her hunger. She had thought that these foods were helping her, but in Syndrome X, high GI carbohydrates will increase the appetite.

Over a 6-month period Maggie lost 17 kilograms and also considerably reduced her potbelly. She was able to fit into her old clothes and wear attractive belts again.

I find that many overweight women are taking inappropriate Hormone Replacement Therapy, which is aggravating their weight problem. It is not wise to take tablets containing strong or synthetic hormones, as these will increase the workload of the liver. I recommend hormone creams or patches containing natural oestrogen and progesterone, as these are absorbed directly through the skin and bypass the liver. If we can reduce the workload of the liver it will be a more efficient fat burning organ.

John's Case History

John was undergoing treatment for male menopause (andropause) and was receiving injections of testosterone every 6 weeks. He was a busy man with his own business, and did not have much time to exercise or relax. He was apple shaped with abdominal obesity and a waist to hip ratio of 1.3.

John had the chemical imbalances of Syndrome X with elevated triglycerides, LDL cholesterol and fasting insulin levels. His high blood pressure was controlled with anti-hypertensive medication and he also took cholesterol-lowering drugs. At the age of 49 he found that the drug side effects were really destroying his sex life and slowing him down, so that his enjoyment of life was decreasing. He was frustrated especially as he had been told that the testosterone injections were going to make him feel wonderful. Indeed the injections had helped him initially, but his increasing weight and the drug side effects were negating the short-lived benefits of the testosterone injections.

I started John on the Syndrome X eating plan, so that he had low-fat protein at every meal and greatly increased his consumption of raw foods and vegetables. He stopped drinking diet sodas and started drinking water. He was allowed 3 cups of black coffee daily, as he really enjoyed his coffee. If he became hungry in between meals, he was allowed to nibble on the Syndrome X snack pack, or eat a can of seafood. As a big man he had a huge appetite, so that healthy snacks were vital to see him through. I also recommended a powerful liver tonic and a nutritional supplement to reduce his insulin resistance.

I stopped his testosterone injections and checked his blood levels of testosterone and DHEA, 3 months later. His levels were found to be at the lower limit of normal, so I prescribed a cream containing a combination of testosterone 10mg and DHEA 20mg daily.

Over a six month period, John lost 27 kilograms and his waist to hip ratio normalised at 0.9. His blood pressure and cholesterol levels also normalised, so that we were able to stop the medications he was taking. This was a great relief to John, as he hated the side effects and wanted to have a normal sex life again. He found that the hormone creams really helped him greatly, and did not produce the on-off effect that the injections had produced. He told me that he looked and felt 20 years younger, and his teenage son was delighted that his father was able to play sports with him once again. His wife was also very pleased to have her husband back, as she said, with “the old twinkle in his eyes!”

17

Chapter Seventeen

Assessing your body weight

Assessing your body weight

Simply by looking in the mirror it can be difficult to judge just how overweight or underweight you are. Perhaps you would prefer not to know!

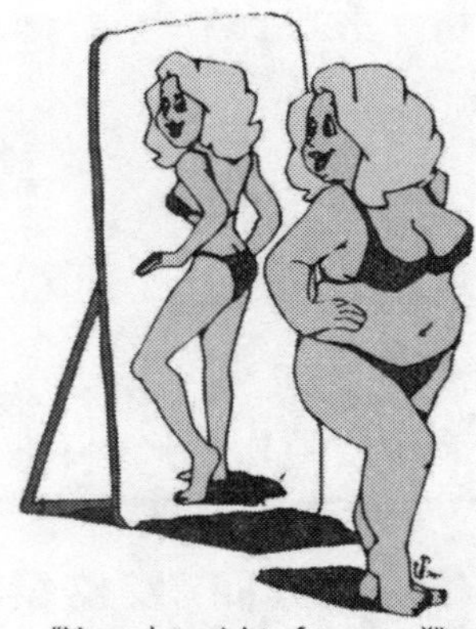

"Never lose sight of your goal!"

A useful graphic way of representing your weight can be done by plotting your weight (along the vertical axis), alongside your height (along the horizontal axis) on the weight for height graph below.

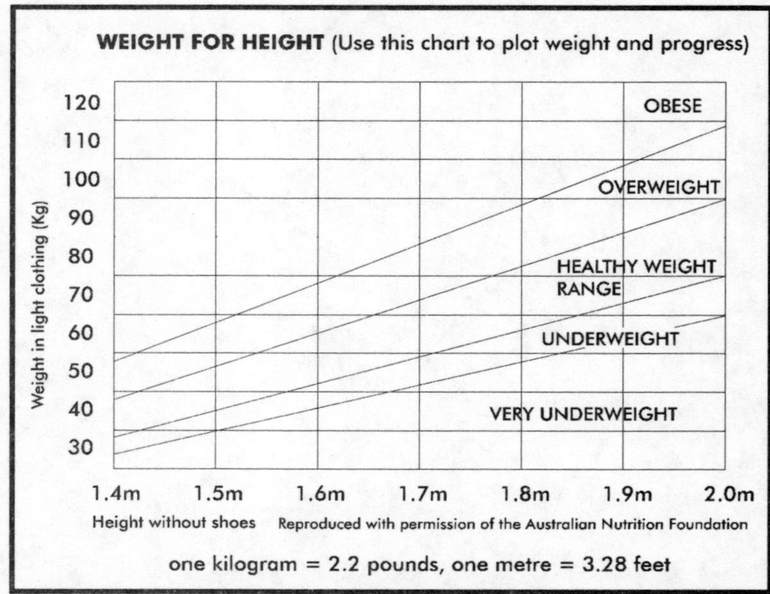

Body Mass Index (BMI)

A useful way of assessing your body weight is a ratio known as the Body Mass Index (BMI). For those not good at maths don't tune out, as it is really very simple! You can calculate your Body Mass Index by dividing your weight (in kilograms) by the square of your height (in metres).

$$\textbf{BMI} = \frac{\text{weight (kilograms)}}{\text{height x height (metres)}}$$

For example if you weigh 75 kilograms and are 1.69 metres (169 centimetres) tall then your

$$\textbf{BMI} = \frac{\text{75 kilograms}}{\text{1.69 x 1.69 metres}}$$

$$= \frac{75}{2.856}$$

Your BMI= 26.26

Note:

To convert pounds to kilograms, divide the pounds by 2.2 – for example 154 pounds divided by 2.2 = 70kilograms

To convert inches to metres, multiply the inches by 0.0254 – for example 68 inches multiplied by 0.0254 = 1.727 metres.

If you don't like equations, you can easily work out your BMI from the scale on the following page.

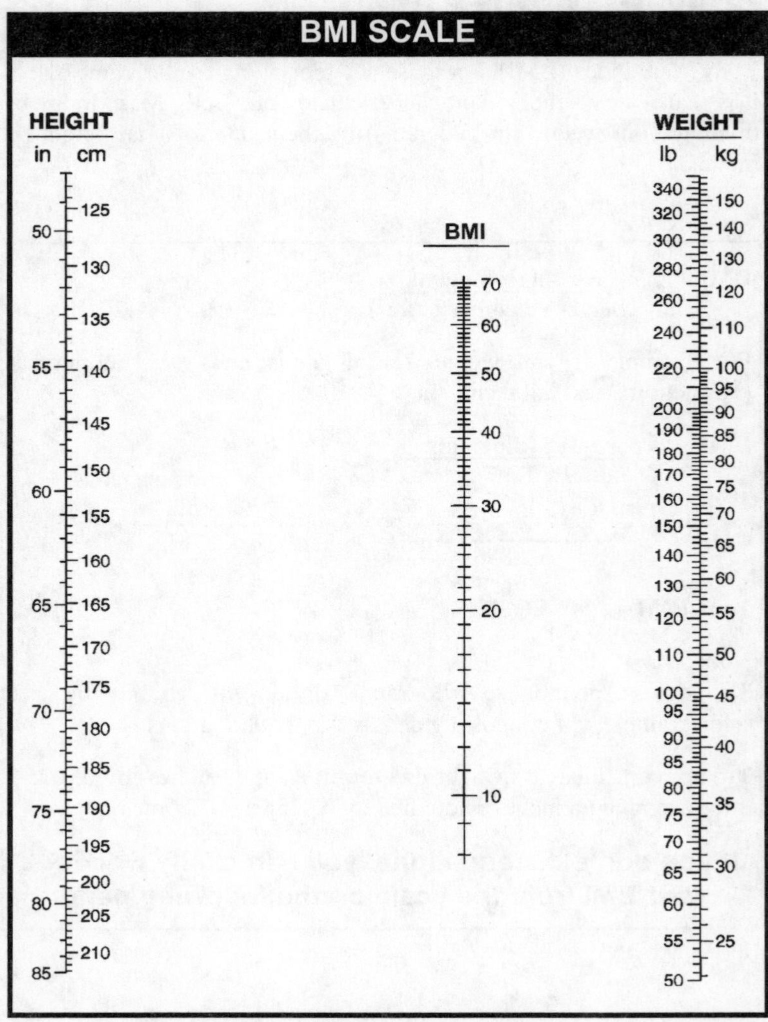

To use the scale, place a ruler between your weight (undressed) and your height (without shoes). Then read your BMI on the middle scale.

BMI Scale

BMI less than 16	= lean to underweight
BMI 19 to 25	= desirable for women
BMI 20 to 26	= desirable for men
BMI 26 to 30	= overweight
BMI 30 to 40	= obesity
BMI over 40	= severe obesity

When weighing yourself choose the same time of the day, wearing no clothes.

Weight can vary by 1-2 kilograms over one day, due to fluid retention, constipation, a full bladder, exercise and hormonal changes. Thus weighing yourself once or twice a week is sufficient, less frustrating and less prone to small errors.

What should the body fat percentage of your total body weight be?

AGE	PERCENTAGE BODY FAT
Women	
Up to 30 years	20 to 26%
31 to 40 years	21 to 27%
41 to 50 years	22 to 28%
Over 50 years	22 to 31%
Men	
Up to 30 years	12 to 18%
31 to 40 years	13 to 19%
Over 40 years	13 to 21%

Note: Women whose body fat percentage falls below 15% will have problems with their body's production of sex hormones. This can cause infertility and lead to absent menstruation and osteoporosis.

18

Chapter Eighteen

Obstacles to Successful Weight Loss

Obstacles to Successful Weight Loss

1. Weight Loss Plateaus

My eating plan provides both men and women with a very high success rate in long-term weight loss and weight control. It is healthy, nutritionally balanced and easy to follow. You will not be hungry, as the foods are not low in fat or protein, and contain slowly digested carbohydrates. If you feel hungry while on the Syndrome X eating plan you should eat. Choose the healthy foods and snacks mentioned in this book to satisfy your own natural hunger.

Over many years I have come to realise that restrictive diets that are very low in fat and calories never work for very long. It is impossible to make these semi-starvation diets a way of life – they are just too hard and make you feel deprived. It is not a "low-food diet" that you want, it is a "right-food eating plan" that you can enjoy and live with.

I am often surprised by the unrealistic expectations of those who are trying to lose weight. They expect to lose all their weight within a month, and then to keep it off permanently just by reducing calories. The problem is that with very low-fat low-calorie diets your metabolism slows right down, and when you start to eat "normally" again, the lost weight is regained more rapidly than it was lost. So in desperation you start the diet again, which further slows down your metabolism and you put on even more weight than you carried before. This leads to the phenomena of the "yoyo dieter", who after a lifetime of misery and starvation, ends up fatter than they were when they first started dieting.

So I will opt for a gradual steady weight loss every time, rather than a super quick loss of body fat.

Now it is time to mention the phenomena of the "weight loss plateau", which can affect every sensible dieter and is really not to be feared. The "weight loss plateau" can be described as a flattening out in the weight loss curve while following a diet or eating plan. During this flattening of the curve, weight loss ceases for a variable period of time from 2 weeks up to 6 weeks. This is the dangerous time when many people become frustrated and falsely believe that the eating plan they are following is not working. You are wrong it is working! During this plateau phase, the desired changes in your liver and metabolism are still happening, even though you cannot see them.

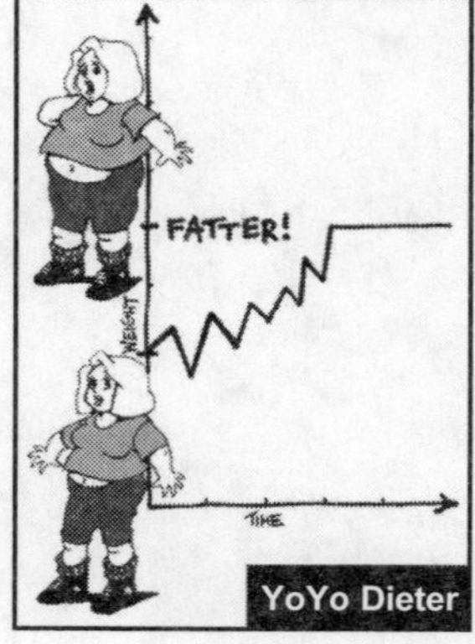

YoYo Dieter

For example it takes time to -

- Reduce insulin levels and improve insulin resistance.
- Remove the unhealthy fat from the liver, and turn your liver into an efficient fat burner, and not a fat storing organ.
- Balance your hormones.

All this will be happening while you are following my eating plan and using appropriate supplements, but you will not see these things occurring behind the scenes. While your body is busy achieving this metabolic correction, there may be times where weight loss stops, but this is only temporary. Indeed these are necessary lulls in your rate of weight loss. If you become impatient and revert to eating all the high GI carbohydrates and unhealthy fats during a plateau phase, you will undo weeks of beneficial changes, not to mention your own hard work. Indeed by jumping off the eating plan while in a plateau phase, you may become a yoyo dieter. So my message is just hang in there! The desired changes are happening inside your liver and your fat cells, and within a few weeks weight loss will resume at a normal healthy pace.

If you do fall off the wagon, do not freak out and lose your inspiration. Just get back onto the eating plan, but remember it may take a few weeks before you see the weight coming off. However your energy levels should improve within a few days of recommencing the eating plan in this book.

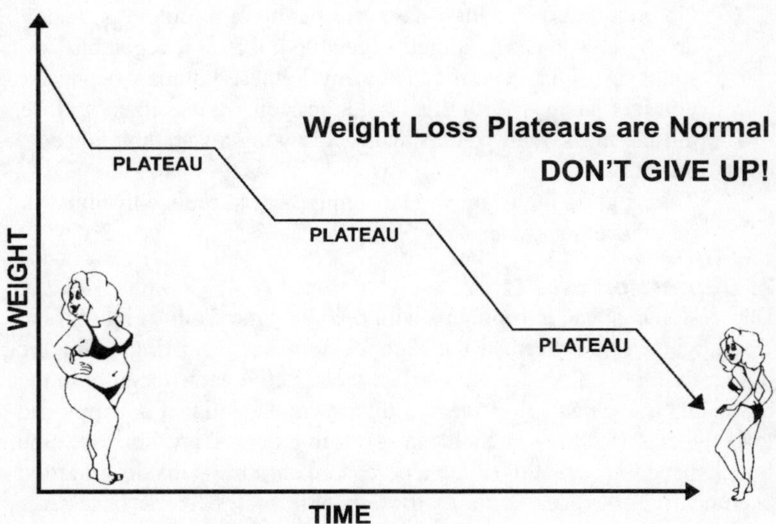

Some people have been overweight for many years, and find it extremely difficult to commence losing weight, or find themselves in a plateau of no weight loss for too long. If this is you and you are becoming impatient there are several things that you can try –

- For 3 to 4 weeks just have meals comprised of lean red meat, eggs or seafood, combined with salad vegetables and/or cooked green leafy vegetables. Avoid all starchy vegetables such as potato, carrots, swede and pumpkin. This diet is virtually free of carbohydrate and will put you into a state of fat burning or ketosis. Your insulin levels will plummet and after several days you will not feel hungry. Those with diabetes or kidney disease are not able to follow this strict regime.
- Go on a vegetable juice fast for 4 days. You can dilute the juices with 50% water to improve kidney function. Your body will go into a state of fat burning and you will probably have ketones in your urine by day 2 of the juice fast. The presence of ketones in the urine indicates that you are breaking down your body fat and using it for energy. *See page 111.* This state of ketosis is only temporary and is not a problem as long as you are not diabetic, or suffer with kidney disease or heart failure. Always check with your own doctor to see if it is safe for you to try a juice fast.
- Go on a liquid diet for 7 days, consisting of a protein powder drink *(see page 216),* diluted vegetable juices and vegetable soups or broths. You may have any of these liquids whenever you feel hungry. With this liquid diet you are less likely to lose muscle mass, than you are while following a vegetable juice only fast.
- Take a good liver tonic and a supplement to reduce insulin resistance – *see page 53*

2. Depression and Stress

Depression can lead to problems with body weight, from weight loss to weight gain. This is because the chemical imbalance existing within the brain of depressed people, may affect the appetite control centre in the brain. Of course just being overweight may make you feel unhappy and lower your self-esteem, which can result in a depressive illness. Some people need to overeat to fill up a perceived emptiness inside, and food becomes their solace. Some of these people may become obsessive-compulsive eaters.

If you feel that depression and stress may be sabotaging your weight loss efforts you can look into several options –

- Support groups such as Over-Eaters Anonymous can be very helpful.
- Join a club with physical activities such as a tennis club, bushwalking club or a swimming club. Aqua-aerobics can be the best exercise for overweight persons, as it does not stress the joints.
- Have a regular therapeutic massage to relieve pent up physical and emotional stresses.
- Go for a walk each morning with a group of friends.
- Seek regular counselling from a psychotherapist or psychologist to work on the subconscious reasons why you crave comfort foods in excess amounts.
- If the depression is severe enough for your doctor to classify it as a "clinical depression" you may need to take anti-depressant medication.

There are basically 3 types of anti-depressant drugs –

- The Tricyclic anti-depressant drugs – these are helpful to reduce anxiety and panic attacks, improve sleep and alleviate depression. However in some people they can increase the appetite, which may lead to weight gain. Thus you really need to stick with the Syndrome X eating plan if you are taking Tricyclic anti-depressants.
- The Serotonin Re-uptake Inhibitors (SRI's) and the Selective Serotonin Re-uptake Inhibitors (SSRI's). These drugs can have a variable effect upon weight, however in the majority of cases do not cause significant weight gain. Indeed in some people with clinical depression, they may help with weight loss.
- The Monoamine Oxidase Inhibitors (MAOI's) are effective anti-depressants that often help with weight loss. The newer drugs such as the Selective Monoamine Oxidase Inhibitors are safer than the older drugs, and an effective example of these is Aurorix.

3. Hypoglycaemia and trigger foods

Hypoglycaemia or low blood sugar, is a common cause of strong cravings for sweets and high GI carbohydrates. Thus it is important to prevent hypoglycaemia. To avoid hypoglycaemia you need to ensure that you are eating first class protein at least 3 times daily. If you are busy, you can use a protein powder drink, protein snacks such as canned seafood, and nuts and seeds. Tasty nuts are macadamias, pecans, walnuts, and Brazil nuts, which are convenient, and have a significant amount of satisfying healthy fats compared to pure carbohydrates. For this reason they tend to suppress the appetite. Nuts are low in carbohydrate and have a very low GI index, which will help to prevent erratic fluctuations in blood sugar levels.

Avocados are also excellent to eat if you have a craving for excessive carbohydrates. Avocadoes are high in mono-unsaturated fats, and low in carbohydrate, with a very low GI. Foods high in mono-unsaturated fats have been shown to reduce insulin resistance. Avocados are healthy and filling, and are delicious if you fill their cavity with seafood. They also taste very nice with sun-dried tomatoes and olives, which are very low GI foods.

If you must have something sweet try eating fruit, the Syndrome X Snack Pack, or using the herb Stevia as a natural sweetener.

What do you do if you get cravings for the wrong foods?

The taste of foods high in carbohydrate and sugar can be addictive, especially if you have severe drops in your blood sugar levels. Once you become accustomed to eating these high sugar foods again, your body will come to expect them regularly, so it is best to stop as soon as possible.

Sometimes the cravings for sweets can become overbearing and you need to have some strategies to overcome these cravings.

To reduce cravings I recommend –

- Use a protein powder designed for Syndrome X *(see page 216)* when you get a craving. The full range of amino acids in this powder will help to stabilise blood sugar levels and increase energy. The supplemental L - glutamine in the powder can act as a fuel for the brain and reduce the fatigue associated with fluctuations in blood sugar. This protein powder also contains supplemental chromium picolinate, which helps the Glucose Tolerance Factor to stabilise blood sugar levels. Simply mix the protein powder in water or non-dairy milk, and make a shake in the blender.

- The craving for sugar and refined carbohydrates can often be replaced with salty foods. For example, you could try high protein bread, or sourdough bread, drizzled with cold pressed olive oil and vegemite, sardines or anchovies, sun dried tomatoes and olives with low fat fetta cheese.

Addiction to chocolate

Some people need chocolate more than love and cannot exist without any chocolate in their lives. In all honesty I cannot think of a substitute for the experience of chocolate. I recently met a woman who suffered with obesity and Syndrome X, and consumed seven family sized blocks of chocolate a week!

Although chocolate has a relatively low GI, it is still very high in fat and calories. If you are a chocolate addict and must have chocolate, I suggest that you allow your self to have chocolate once a week as a treat, but do not eat the family size block and stick to a small chocolate bar.

4. Lack of Exercise

We all know that regular exercise will assist in increasing the metabolic rate and weight loss. However some people don't enjoy exercise and prefer to watch someone else do it. Furthermore if you are overweight, you may feel uncomfortable about wearing a swim suit or exercise shorts, or mixing with slim people at the local gym. One thing that I have found easy to do is to put on some music at home and dance around the lounge room. You can also exercise with a small pair of hand weights while you dance, or follow along with an exercise video, in the privacy of your own home. The hand weights will tone and firm the arms, which may become flabby with weight loss. Some people find it useful to acquire the help of a personal trainer, although this can be expensive. Your exercise routine should be done every day to gradually improve your fitness level.

If you fall into the very over-weight range, the best exercise to start with is gentle swimming or walking. As you lose weight, more strenuous exercises such as aerobics or jogging can be started.

Be on the look-out for opportunities to exercise, such as getting off the bus a few stops earlier, taking the stairs instead of the elevator, leaving your car at home, or stopping for a walk in the park at lunch breaks. Some days you may feel like putting it off, but try to force yourself to overcome laziness because the results are many times worth the effort. The more you exercise the better you will look and feel. If you burn up 250 calories (1050 kJ) daily with exercise, this would result in a weekly weight loss of 230grams (0.23 kg). If you burn up 500 calories (2100 kJ) daily with exercise, this would result in a weekly weight loss of 500grams (1/2kg).

ACTIVITY	CALORIES BURNED PER MINUTE
VERY LIGHT e.g. dusting slow walking, yoga	**2 (8.4kJ)**
MODERATE e.g. brisk walking energetic gardening scrubbing the floor	**3.5-7 (14.7-29.4kJ)**
HEAVY e.g. running, aerobics swimming laps, rowing weight training	**>7.5 (>31.5kJ)**

Exercises for Cellulite

Exercise used as part of a program to reduce cellulite and help to keep it off needs to be isotonic. This means it needs to take you through a broad range of large movements such as in cycling, swimming, running, power walking or rowing. This kind of exercise shortens and lengthens your muscles rhythmically. You need to become fit all over, that is why aerobic exercise, especially the low-impact type, is extremely beneficial for cellulite. The fitter you are the lower your resting heart rate is, which means you can deal better with stress, without such a large build-up of chemical by-products in your system. The best exercise is definitely a constant rhythmical type, where you are using the large muscle groups at an intensity that increases your heart rate to 60 per cent of your maximum heart rate. This is called your target heart rate. It is necessary to achieve your target heart rate, if you want to increase your metabolic rate, and so increase the rate at which you burn up excess fat.

To find your **maximum heart rate**, subtract your age from 220.

To find your **target heart** rate, multiply the above figure (220 minus your age) by 0.6.

For example, if you are 40 years old, your maximum heart rate = 220 minus 40 = 180 beats per minute.

Your target heart rate = 180 x 0.6 = 108 beats per minute.

By reaching your target heart rate during exercise, you will increase your metabolic rate.

To reduce cellulite you should leave no longer than 24 hours between each session of exercise. You can work out for anything between fifteen to sixty minutes a session, three to five times a week. Ideally, you could do five, thirty-minute sessions per week, as that would keep your metabolic rate up and running, therefore preventing the build up of cellulite.

Massage and hydrotherapy are also excellent in helping to stimulate lymphatic drainage and reduce cellulite.

During exercise, skeletal muscle needs carbohydrate, and gets it by converting glucose or glycogen to lactate. This is a very effective way to burn calories. In sedentary people skeletal muscle cells demonstrate insulin resistance, and exercise can help to reduce insulin resistance.

Exercise will improve the health of your heart and lungs, regulate your desire for food and speed up your weight loss.

Colin's Case history

Colin was a typical example of a man who was addicted to carbohydrates. He started his day with black coffee laden with 3 teaspoons of sugar, and tried to avoid eating, as he thought this would help him to lose weight. He then went to his office job and found that by 11am he started to crave something sweet. He went to the snack machine where he obtained a diet soda and a candy bar. He said the sugar tasted great going down, but once it hit his stomach he felt nauseated.

Lunchtime consisted of more diet sodas and a large plate of pasta covered with a creamy sauce. The pasta gave him a big dose of carbohydrate and filled him up until around 3pm. By this time he needed more coffee laden with sugar and a sweet biscuit. On his way home from work he thought of sugar and knew every snack bar on the way home from work. He could not resist the temptation to buy some sugary donuts and more diet soda. By 7pm he felt exhausted, and usually made himself a quick meal of toast and jam or toast and cheese. His diet was very poor, being deficient in protein, vegetables and essential fatty acids.

Colin felt quite hopeless about losing weight and had tried everything from stomach stapling to laxatives, emetics and many low-fat low-calorie diets. He believed it was his fault and that he would never be able to lose his addiction to carbohydrates.

When Colin came to see me he was 130 kilograms (286 pounds) and was 1.75 metres (5 foot 10 inches) tall. He had a lot of weight accumulated around his trunk and abdominal area, and a roll of fat around the upper abdomen. His legs were reasonably slim and muscular, and his hips were narrow. He really had upper level body obesity, and was the Android Body Type *(see page 166).*

Blood tests revealed that Colin had Syndrome X, as his fasting triglycerides, LDL cholesterol and insulin levels were all elevated. A 3-hour Glucose Tolerance test showed that he had temporarily elevated levels of blood glucose, which then became abnormally low after 3 hours. At this time he had a marked craving for sugar and felt weak and shaky.

I explained to Colin that he had a chemical imbalance known as Syndrome X, which was 90% of the reason that he was addicted to carbohydrates and refined-sugar. He was relieved to know that there was a medical problem that made him crave the wrong foods, and also kept him too exhausted to exercise.

I started Colin on the Syndrome X diet so that he was having regular protein. He began having eggs for breakfast, a large salad and chicken for lunch, and seafood and vegetables with salad for his evening meal. While he was at work he kept a supply of raw nuts and seeds and his Syndrome - X protein powder handy. He would use these things to snack on when the sugar cravings hit him.

This gave Colin more confidence, as he now had a very specific way of eating to put himself back in control of his body. After the first week he phoned me, saying that he had not lost any weight but felt much more energetic and had not had one craving for sugar. Indeed he was wondering if he was eating too much, as the salads and vegetables took much longer to eat than his previous foods, and really seemed to fill him up. After the second week he started to lose weight steadily from his abdomen, and lost the bloated feeling he had always had around his abdomen. One thing he found very handy to stave off carbohydrate cravings was canned crabmeat. He took cans of crabmeat to work, and ate one can in the mid-afternoon, which kept him craving-free until his evening meal. He loved the taste of crabmeat and thought it was a real treat being able to eat shellfish as he desired. For years he had thought that he must avoid shellfish, as it would raise his cholesterol levels. Little did he know that cholesterol like this in its natural form, combined with pure protein was a great weapon against his chemical imbalance. Indeed it was sugar and refined carbohydrates that were causing his metabolic problem, and not protein or pure cholesterol.

In total Colin lost 38 kilograms over 18 months, and it all came off from his abdomen and trunk area. An ultrasound scan of his liver showed that it was no longer fatty and his blood tests were now all normal. He no longer had Syndrome X. Now that his body chemistry was back to normal, he no longer craved refined carbohydrates and sugar, which to him was utterly amazing. When he became hungry he thought of protein and vegetables. He also enjoyed the flavour of the protein powder, which he used regularly to keep his energy levels high.

19

Chapter Nineteen

Diet Tips for Losing Weight

Diet Tips for Losing Weight

Slimming Protein Powder for Syndrome X

Protein powders can provide a source of complete protein in a convenient and easily digested form. They are great for a quick energy burst, and to sustain you during hunger pangs in between meals. If you are busy, or just feeling lazy, you can make a complete meal out of a protein powder, and some fruit or vegetables.

I have found that whey protein concentrate is the most effective protein supplement for those with a weight problem or Syndrome X. Soy protein is not such a high quality protein as whey protein concentrate is. Those allergic to whole dairy products will not usually have a problem with whey protein, as it is very easy to digest.

I prefer protein powders that are unsweetened, or sweetened with the natural herb Stevia, rather than artificially sweetened powders.

You should look for a protein powder that contains the following ingredients –

- Whey protein concentrate as its main ingredient.
- Extra amounts of the amino acid Taurine, which is essential for healthy liver function and fat metabolism– *see page 72*
- Extra amounts of the amino acid Glutamine, which can act as a fuel for the brain, and reduces cravings for sweets and alcohol. It is also useful for digestive disorders. Laboratory studies in mice have shown that supplemental glutamine is of benefit in glucose control and in reducing elevated insulin levels - *REF. 32.* Glutamine reduces the levels of blood fats and reduces insulin resistance. Glutamine is also able to increase lean muscle mass and decrease the body fat percentage, probably by its beneficial effect upon blood glucose control.
- Added chromium picolinate, which helps to reduce insulin resistance and stabilise blood sugar levels.

Avoid protein powders containing added sugar or sugar substitutes such as maltodextrin as these can have a high GI.

This protein powder can be used in the following ways –

- To make a pleasant drink by itself in between meals, or as an accompaniment to fresh fruit pieces or muesli for breakfast

- To make a "smoothie" with added fruit (such as banana, strawberries or blackberries etc.) and ground flaxseed in a blender. You can add a raw egg if you want even more protein and are using the "smoothie" to replace a meal.
- To make a tropical "smoothie" on a hot summer day – try adding some coconut milk or coconut cream, small amounts of fresh fruits (such as kiwi fruit, mango, papaya or banana), a few drops of vanilla essence – blend all together in blender and serve on the rocks – delicious!
- To sprinkle over cereals or desserts to increase their protein content.

For more information about first class protein call the Health Advisory Service on 02 4655 8855

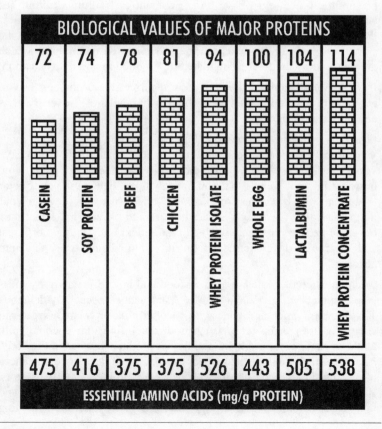

BIOLOGICAL VALUES OF MAJOR PROTEINS

	CASEIN	SOY PROTEIN	BEEF	CHICKEN	WHEY PROTEIN ISOLATE	WHOLE EGG	LACTALBUMIN	WHEY PROTEIN CONCENTRATE
Biological value	72	74	78	81	94	100	104	114
ESSENTIAL AMINO ACIDS (mg/g PROTEIN)	475	416	375	375	526	443	505	538

Should I avoid Eggs and Coconut to reduce cholesterol?

Eggs are high in cholesterol and if we listen to some nutritionists and the popular press we often find that eggs are portrayed as dangerous and unhealthy, especially for those with heart problems. I do not agree with the general opinion that eggs should be considered suspect, because eggs contain high concentrations of many valuable nutrients. Moreover most of the studies that showed eggs raised cholesterol were done using powdered eggs. Powdered eggs contain oxidised or damaged cholesterol known as oxy-cholesterol, and this has a different effect in the body than pure fresh cholesterol. Other studies have found that hard-boiled eggs do not raise cholesterol levels in the majority of patients. A study done at the University of California found that the consumption of two boiled eggs daily did not increase cholesterol levels. The reason why eggs consumed in moderation is health promoting, is that eggs have a high content of lecithin. Lecithin has been proven to lower cholesterol and helps to keep it soluble, so that it does not form plaques in the blood vessels. Eggs are also high in the sulphur bearing amino acids taurine, cysteine and methionine, which are required by the liver to regulate bile production and detoxification.

Eggs are only healthy if they are cooked correctly, and the best way to eat them is poached, boiled, scrambled or in omelettes. Never fry eggs and only use fresh eggs.

Generally speaking I would say limit the ingestion of eggs to no more than 12 to 15 per week, however this is an individual thing. If you have very high cholesterol, you should ask your doctor to guide you, however I do not believe that you must avoid all eggs. Ask your doctor to do a fasting blood test to check the effect of eating eggs in your particular case. This way you can be sure and prove what effect they have. Remember that everyone is an individual with unique hormonal and metabolic differences, and nutritional medicine takes this into account.

Coconut is another much maligned food and indeed is unworthy of its jaded reputation. I personally prefer Asian sauces, especially delicious Thai recipes, which are made with coconut milk or coconut cream, to creamy sauces made with dairy products. I find that coconut milk and/or cream sauces are light, and do not produce mucous in the body. I have never found that fresh coconut, coconut milk or coconut sauces have caused high cholesterol levels or weight problems in my patients. If you have a fatty liver it is important not to overindulge in any fat and this is just common sense. Simply consume a sensible and satisfying amount of these foods, and make sure that they are fresh, so that their contained fats are not oxidised. Remember that the liver makes 80% of the body's cholesterol, and cholesterol levels are regulated automatically by a HEALTHY liver. If you consume a little more cholesterol on one day, the liver will not manufacture as much of its own cholesterol, and things will balance out nicely. Liver function has a much greater effect upon cholesterol levels, than does a modest consumption of healthy foods containing cholesterol.

Can I eat a lot of dairy products on this program?

I have purposely excluded all dairy products, from the recipes in this book, except for a small amount of fetta or Parmesan cheese, and plain yogurt. This is because of my personal beliefs and experiences and also because of the influence of several books I have read on the subject of cow's milk. My dietary philosophies are not completely conventional as far as many dieticians and nutritionists are concerned, and will not be accepted by all.

I have found that everyone is different, with unique hormonal and metabolic characteristics, which means that some people will have individual intolerances to foods. This means that some trial and error will be involved in finding the best diet for oneself. Some people are able to consume dairy products with no problems. Others will have problems from eating dairy products, such as recurrent infections of the respiratory tract, sinuses, ears and skin, mucous excess, different types of allergic reactions, asthma, and irritable bowel. I have found that in some people, dairy products aggravate autoimmune diseases such as primary biliary cirrhosis and autoimmune hepatitis. Dairy products may also aggravate cysts and lumps in the thyroid and breasts and granulomatous diseases such as sarcoidosis. I have found that in those with chronic or recurrent viral infections of the lymphatic system, such as glandular fever, it is necessary to eliminate all dairy products from the diet. These recommendations are based upon my own clinical experiences and not everyone will have had these same experiences, or indeed will agree with my recommendations. It is up to you to make up your own mind and if you have any of the above problems you may decide to follow the recipes and way of eating espoused in this book. The "proof of the pudding is in the eating", so why not try it for 4 to 6 months, although 12 months is better, and see if there is a change in your health? Dairy products consist of animal milks and their derivatives, namely butter, cheese, cream, yoghurt, icecream and dairy chocolate.

Calcium Rich Foods Table

Food	Amount	Calcium (mg)
Seafood		
Salmon (canned)	1 cup	431
Oysters, raw	1 cup	226
Sardines (with bones)	100gms(3.6oz)	300
Tuna (with bones)	100gms(3.6oz)	290
Fish (fresh, cooked)	100gms(3.6oz)	35
Legumes		
Tofu	112 gms(4oz)	80-150
Tempeh	112 gms(4oz)	172
Chickpeas	1 cup (cooked)	150
Tortillas, corn	2	120
Black beans	1 cup (cooked)	135
Soy milk (unfortified)	1 cup	60
Soy milk (fortified)	1 cup	300
Dairy		
Cows Milk (whole)	1 cup	288
Cows Milk (skim)	1 cup	300
Goats milk	1 cup	295
Cheese (cheddar,Swiss)	42 gms(1.5oz)	300
Cottage cheese	1 cup	150
Feta cheese	28 gms(1oz)	129
Yoghurt	1 cup	294
Nuts and Seeds		
Brazil nuts	1 cup	260
Sunflower seeds (hulled)	1 cup	174
Sesame seeds (ground)	3 tablespoons	300
Almonds (hulled)	1 cup	300
Tahini (sesame paste)	1 tablespoon	85
Sea Vegetables (cooked)		
Wakame	1 cup	520
Agar-agar	1 cup	400
Kelp (kombu)	1 cup	305
Hijiki	1 cup	610
Dulse (dry)	1 cup	567
Green Vegetables (cooked)		
Parsley (raw)	1 cup	122
Bok choy	1 cup	200
Spinach	1 cup	178
Broccoli	1 cup	100
Beet greens	1 cup	165
Watercress (raw)	1 cup	53
Rhubarb	1 cup	348
Collard greens	1 cup	300
Dandelion greens	1 cup	147

As you can see, many different food groups contain calcium, such as green leafy vegetables, seeds, nuts and fish. One of the highest calcium sources comes from sea vegetables (seaweeds), so popular in many Asian cultures, especially Japanese food. It is easy to get all the calcium you need without eating dairy products. All you need to do is have a varied diet, and if necessary take a calcium supplement.

Healthy Foods to eat regularly

- Legumes – any beans, peas, lentils
- Unprocessed cereals and grains
- Raw nuts and seeds
- Fresh vegetables – raw and cooked
- Fresh fruits
- Low fat poultry – skin removed
- All seafood and shellfish
- Eggs – boiled or poached (not fried). Omega-3 enriched eggs have a lot more of the omega-3 fatty acids (ALA & DHA) than regular eggs. These omega-3 enriched eggs come from hens fed on a high omega- 3 diet such as canola and flaxseeds.
- Cold pressed vegetable, nut and seed oils
- Vinegar – apple cider, Balsamic, organic, wine vinegars
- Avocados and olives
- Fresh herbs and spices

Healthy foods to eat in moderation

- Lean fresh red meat
- Low GI pasta
- Spreads made with nuts, hummus, tahini
- Whole grain breads

Unhealthy foods to avoid

- Fatty meats
- Preserved meats – ham, bacon, sausages, salami, cabanossi, hot dogs, delicatessen meats, luncheon meats, fritz, pizza meats and smoked meats
- Hamburger meat
- Pizza with cheese and preserved meats
- High fat dairy products = cream, cream cheese, ice cream, high fat cheeses and butter
- Deep-fried foods such as French fries, deep-fried chicken nuggets, fried chicken, deep-fried seafood
- Refined carbohydrates – made with white sugar and white flour

- Sweet fizzy drinks – sodas and diet drinks
- Candies, lollies, snack bars, chocolate bars, high in sugar
- Doughnuts, croissants, cakes made with refined sugar and white flour
- Processed foods containing hydrogenated vegetable oils (transfatty acids)
- Margarines containing hydrogenated vegetable oils or trans-fatty acids
- Shortening
- Foods with a lot of pastry such as meat pies and pasties
- Packaged snack foods high in fat, especially hydrogenated oils and trans fatty acids, such as potato chips, pretzels, corn chips, cookies, packaged muffins and cakes
- Foods that are not fresh
- Pickled foods with added sugar
- Fruit juices high in sugar

In particular it is good to avoid foods that combine high GI carbohydrates with high fat, such as ice cream, pretzels, potato chips, many packaged cakes and biscuits, cream cakes, sweet puddings with custard. Foods combining high fat with high GI carbohydrates will cause high insulin levels. The high insulin levels tell our bodies to store fat and not burn fat.

Be careful with so called "low fat" snack foods, as we may be inclined to eat twice as much, which will result in more calories than foods with a normal amount of fat.

Healthy Snacks for Syndrome X

These are to munch when you get unexpectedly hungry and start to crave foods high in sugar, or high GI refined carbohydrates.

Choose from the following selections -

Handful of raw nuts and seeds – these are great for those with Syndrome X because they do not contain too much saturated fat, as their fats are mostly mono- or polyunsaturated. They are also high in fibre and vitamin E.

Fresh fruit - 2 pieces maximum at a time

Fresh crunchy sticks/pieces of celery, carrot, capsicum, broccoli florets, cherry tomatoes with spicy salsa, or fresh avocado dip, or hummus.

One small can of crab meat, salmon or tuna

A handful of fresh prawns

Cold roast meat and chicken slices (remove fat)

Eggs – curried, boiled, poached or made into an omelette with vegetables

Half an avocado filled with crabmeat, or salmon, or tuna

Two Ryvita biscuit or sesame crackers with tomato and salmon, tuna or crabmeat

Ryvita biscuit with olive oil or tahini and sliced vine ripened tomatoes (add black pepper & salt to taste)

Soy yoghurt with fruit (only small amounts)

Raw vegetable juices

If you feel like a cleansing snack – chop up a mixture of raw vegetables (green beans, lettuce, celery, cucumber, cauliflower, broccoli, bok choy, leeks, sprouts, snow peas, carrots, capsicum, etc) and serve with a nice dressing poured over using cold pressed oil, squeeze of lemon, Balsamic or apple cider vinegar, garlic and hummus etc.

Celery sticks with natural peanut butter filling

Synd-X Protein powder smoothie with fresh berries – use water for less carbohydrates

Ryvita with Soy cheese and/or natural peanut butter

Syndrome X Snack Pack containing –

½ cup dried apple chopped

1 cup of mixed almonds & Brazil nuts

½ cup sunflower seeds

½ cup pepitas

½ cup dried apricots

½ cup roasted chickpeas, soybeans or broad beans

½ cup flaked coconut

This pack provides first class protein, fibre and essential fatty acids.

To obtain ready-made snack packs call 02 4655 8855

Acceptable Snacks when eating out ***(only as a special treat)***

All of the above plus –
BBQ chicken with coleslaw
BBQ – mixed grill with salad
Caesar salad (no croutons)
Greek salad with Fetta cheese
Chef's salad
Cauliflower baked with grated Parmesan cheese
Quiche Lorraine (don't eat all the crust)
Eggs Florentine
Steak and eggs
Sandwich – with meat, fish, egg and/or salad filling (no butter or margarine).
Ploughman's lunch
Pancakes with a savoury filling or fruit
Frittata

20

Chapter Twenty

Protein

Protein

First Class Protein

In nutritional terms when we talk about amino acids, we are referring to the twenty amino acids that are required for the synthesis of proteins in the body. Proteins are large molecules required for the formation of body cells, and they facilitate the chemical reactions in the body that are needed to maintain life.

The twenty amino acids that are needed to manufacture the body's proteins are –
Tyrosine, tryptophan, valine, proline, serine, threonine, lysine, phenylalanine, methionine, glycine, histidine, leucine, isoleucine, cysteine, glutamine, glutamic acid, alanine, aspartic acid, asparagine and arginine. There are other amino acids present in the body that are not required for protein synthesis, such as taurine and ornithine.

The twenty amino acids that are required to synthesise proteins in the body fall into 2 categories:

- **Eight essential amino acids** – phenylalanine, leucine, isoleucine, threonine, lysine, valine, tryptophan, and methionine. These are classed as essential, as they must be obtained from the diet and cannot be manufactured by the human body.
- **Twelve non-essential amino acids** – these can be made in the body from other compounds.

A protein food is called "First Class" if it contains all of the eight essential amino acids. A first class protein is often referred to as a complete protein.

Examples of first class proteins are -
Animal meats such as red meat, white meat and poultry
Seafood
Eggs
Dairy products
Whey protein powder - *see page 217*

Foods from the plant kingdom are generally not first class proteins, and these foods need to be combined in specific ways to provide all the eight essential amino acids at one meal.

To derive first class protein from plant foods you need to –
Combine 3 of the following 4 food groups together, at the **SAME MEAL** –

- Legumes (beans, peas, lentils)
- Grains
- Nuts
- Seeds

So for example, by having a meal containing rice (a grain), with chickpeas (a legume), with sesame seeds, you will obtain first class protein. By combining beans (a legume), with barley (a grain), and almonds (a nut), you will obtain first class protein.

Many vegetarians do not take enough care in combining their food groups, and protein deficiency is not uncommon in strict vegans. A vegetarian diet lacking in protein can lead to an over reliance on starchy carbohydrates, which may lead to weight gain and fatigue.

Protein is essential for everyone, and especially for people with Syndrome X, who need to consume first class protein regularly, at least three times a day. It does not have to be in huge amounts, but should provide all the eight essential amino acids. Complete proteins and pure protein foods either by themselves, or when combined with carbohydrate foods, will moderate the rise in blood sugar and insulin levels after a meal. Indeed eating pure protein with vegetables and no carbohydrate will usually not cause any significant rise in post-meal blood sugar or insulin levels. This will reduce hunger in between meals and help in the initial stages of weight loss.

Vegetarians

To cater for vegetarians many of the recipes in this book are free of animal meats and seafood. You do not have to eat meat, poultry or seafood to follow this eating plan or indeed to overcome Syndrome X, however, some people will find it easier to lose weight if they eat some meat, or at least seafood.

If you are a strict vegetarian or vegan, you can substitute the meat in the recipes with tofu, tempeh or grains, legumes, nuts and seeds. As long as you follow our rules for combining at least 3 vegetarian food groups at one meal (as explained above), you will not become deficient in essential amino acids.

Some people are vegetarian for ethical reasons and this must be respected. Some people are wary of eating meat and poultry because of the risk of Mad Cow Disease.

Mad Cow Disease

Mad Cow Disease is the lay term for the disease in cattle known as Bovine Spongiform Encephalopathy (BSE), which is a progressive neurological disorder. The equivalent disease in sheep is called "scrapie."

BSE can be transmitted to humans where it is known as Creutzfeldt-Jakob Disease (CJD). CJD attacks the brain causing emotional problems, memory loss, clumsiness, and severe dementia. It progresses rapidly and is usually fatal. Thankfully Australia is still free of BSE and this is a good situation that must be protected with stringent controls on the farming of animals for human consumption. BSE has arisen in several European countries because of the intensive "factory farming" of animals where cattle are fed stock feed made of the ground up bodies of dead and diseased cattle. The process of grinding up dead animals for stock feed is called "rendering". This type of stock feed is often called "high protein pellets".

The best way to avoid contracting these horrific diseases is to avoid beef that has been raised this way and purchase only grass-fed beef. If these cattle are organically raised they will be free of growth promoting hormones and other toxic substances. This makes a lot of common sense, as cows and sheep are naturally herbivores or vegetarians, and are designed to graze on grass and not on meat.

21

Chapter Twenty One

Syndrome X Shopping List

Syndrome X Shopping List

- **Beans** – There are many varieties such as soybeans, red kidney, pinto, butter, black, adzuki, flageolet, broad, black-eye, Berlotti, cannellini, Garbanzo, etc. Explore your health food store to see the varieties of beans. The best brands of canned beans and peas are those that have only water and salt added. The least additives the better.
  Some suitable brands are, ANNALISA, GOYA, EDEN, GUSTINI, ROSA, VALVERDE, QUICKPULSE, MCKENZIES
- **Lentils & split peas** –red, green, brown, yellow. Lentils will cook in around 40 minutes with no soaking.
- **Chickpeas** – dry or canned. They need to be cooked the same way as beans.
- **Eggs** – Free range, also omega –3 enriched eggs – TEBBUTTS, MANNING FARM, RSPCA
- **Flour** – buckwheat, whole wheat, rice, baisen, soy flour, corn, spelt, arrowroot; ORGRAN, PUREHARVEST, LOTUS, MCKENZIES
- **Grains** - couscous, quinoa, oats, wheat, spelt, amaranth, barley, buck wheat, bulgur (cracked wheat), rye, and rice - brown rice (long or short grain), basmati, red, jasmine, black, wild rice, Japanese rice. Suitable brands are Lotus, Pureharvest
- **Sauces**
  Miso is fermented bean paste and is made from crushed and boiled soybeans, and is usually mixed with a grain such as rice or barley. Light coloured miso is quite sweet whereas the dark and red coloured miso is savoury. It is important not to boil miso, as it can destroy its nutritional properties. Always add miso at the end of cooking. It is available in health food stores and Asian grocers and supermarkets. Miso has a long shelf life – in an airtight container it can last in the refrigerator for one year.
  Tamari, soy sauce, oyster sauce, fish sauce, chilli sauce, tomato paste. Good brands are Spiral, Lotus, Kikkoman – Naturally Brewed

- **Noodles** – Rice (flat or round), vermicelli, bean thread noodles. Suitable brands are Udon, Hokkien, Ramen; Pureharvest, Arrowhead Mills, Mr Lees, Bamboo Pot, Lotus, Orgran.

- **Oils** – purchase cold pressed oils such as extra virgin olive oil, wheat germ, canola, sunflower, safflower, peanut, flaxseed, mustard seed, grape seed, sesame, walnut, macadamia nut, and soybean oil. Store your oils in dark coloured bottles, with a tight lid, in a cool dark place. Cold pressed oils are preferable because the oil is extracted from the olive, the seed or nut, by mechanical pressing without the use of solvents or heat, which may damage the oils. Cold pressed oils are much higher in anti-oxidants than are processed oils.

- **Salt** – Celtic, vegetable, herb, rock, sea salt or Gomasio, which is a combination of sesame seeds and rock salt.

- **Seafood** – canned sardines, tuna, crabmeat, salmon (pink & red), mackerel, herring. Fresh fish of all varieties and squid (calamari) and shell fish of all varieties.

- **Seaweed** – arame, kombu, nori, wakame and kudzu. Seaweed is used extensively in Japanese cuisine. It has many health benefits including its ability to lower cholesterol, and is very high in trace minerals. It is also helpful for those with sluggish metabolism and thyroid gland problems. Seaweeds are definitely an effective slimming aid.

- **Nuts & Seeds** – pinenuts, walnuts, cashews, macadamias, and Brazil nuts, hazelnuts, almonds, pecans and peanuts. Sunflower seeds, sesame seeds, pumpkinseeds (pepitas) and flaxseed. Nuts and seeds can be ground in a food processor or coffee grinder into a fine powder, which tastes delicious and can be stored in the fridge in an airtight jar. The powder can be added to breakfast cereals, breads and muffins, and sprinkled over fruit for breakfast or desserts. Many people with irritable bowel syndrome and diverticulitis find that they can eat finely groundnuts and seeds without any problems, whereas whole nuts and seeds may aggravate their bowel problems. Nuts and seeds have a very low GI.

- **Sprouts** – bean, snow pea, alfalfa and pea.
- **Tempeh** – some are flavoured varieties, also there are many brands that have a combination of tofu and tempeh – found in Super markets, health food stores, and Asian groceries.
- **Tofu** (silken or firm) – found in Supermarkets, health food stores and Asian groceries. Suitable brands are Nutrisoy, Earth Star, Super Soy, Soyco, Kingland
- **Spreads and Dips -** Tahini (hulled sesame seed paste), hummus, nut spreads (almond, cashews, Brazil, hazelnuts), natural peanut butter, fresh avocado, olive paste, tomato paste, babaghanoush and chopped eggplant. Spread your bread and crackers with these things instead of butter or margarine – found in Supermarkets, Continental delis, health food stores; Suitable brands are Pureharvest, Spiral
- **Vinegar** - apple cider, Balsamic, umboshi, rice wine vinegar, white & red wine vinegar. It is worth knowing that ingesting lemon juice or vinegar with food can lower blood sugar levels after eating. You do not have to ingest large amounts of vinegar to achieve this effect. It has been found that only one tablespoon of vinegar in a salad dressing, when eaten with a meal can lower blood sugar levels by up to 30%. Thus it is worthwhile using vinegar or lemon juice regularly with meals. Apple cider vinegar is the most beneficial for health of all vinegars. Vinegar, especially apple cider vinegar, can also help to improve weak digestion.
- **Pasta** – whole grain and wheat free brands. Suitable brands are Bio-Italia, Pureharvest, Orgran, Spiral and Casalare.
- **Cereals** - oatmeal, rolled oats, wheat germ, cracked wheat, oat or rice bran, pearl barley, polenta (cornmeal), whole wheat porridge, natural muesli, all-bran with added fibre, shredded wheat. Suitable brands are Arrow head mills, Pure Harvest, Lowan, Anchor, Uncle Toby's
- **MILKS** - unsweetened oat, almond, soy, rice, coconut – suitable brands are Australia's Own, Pureharvest, So Natural
- **MAYONNAISE**; Soy Mayonnaise NORGANIC
- **BREADS** – pumpernickel, whole grain, stone ground,

sprouted wheat bread, whole wheat pita, sourdough, chapati (made from chick pea flour or baisen), corn based tortillas, whole grain breads made with cracked wheat, soy, seeds, oats, rye, barley

- **MEATS** – fresh very lean beef, fresh lean veal and pork, lean lamb (leg, loin chops trimmed of all fat)
- **POULTRY** – lean fresh chicken, turkey – organic if available.
- **VEGETABLES** – fresh green leafy of all varieties, salad greens, carrots, beetroots, sweet potato, new potato, celery, capsicum, onions, garlic, leeks, shallots, radish, ginger root, parsnip, turnip, pumpkin, bok choy, broccoli, green beans, green peas, Brussels sprouts, cabbage, cauliflower, spinach, artichokes, zucchini, sweet corn, olives, avocado, cucumber, asparagus, eggplant, parsley, coriander, basil and other fresh herbs. Choose many varieties of vegetables with different colours. Roasted peppers and capsicums, roasted eggplant, marinated vegetables. Tomatoes (fresh and sun dried) and tomato puree (canned).

  Asian vegetables

  Lotus root is available in most Asian groceries and some health food stores. It can be bought dried, frozen or fresh. If you buy it dried, soak it in hot water for 10 minutes, keep the liquid for cooking and continue as per recipe. If you are lucky enough to get it fresh, choose the ones with unblemished skin, peel, slice (approx 0.5cm thick) and place in acidulated water (water with a bit of lemon juice) to prevent them from discolouring. Their taste is quite sweet and the texture crunchy. It will remain crunchy when cooked. They are delicious and the wagon wheel shape adds a beautiful look to your dishes.

  Galangal – tastes like sour ginger, and also similar in looks to ginger. Peel and slice, as you would ginger. Often found in Thai, Malaysian and Indonesian dishes. Has a similar uplifting affect like ginger.

  Shiitake Mushrooms - These Japanese mushrooms are available either fresh (used within a day or two), or dried (can be kept indefinitely in a jar). The fresh mushrooms are firm and dry unlike the field mushroom, which is quite moist. The stems are too tough to eat but are great to use for flavour in stocks. To prepare the dried mushrooms, soak in warm water for 30 minutes, remove the stalks, strain and use the liquid for stocks or soups. To prepare fresh mushrooms, wipe the cap, remove the stalks and use according to the recipe. They are a great source of potassium and fibre and are beneficial for the immune system. Exotic mushrooms can be bought from either Asian grocers or health food stores and some green grocers.

- **SPICES** – chilli (powder, paste or fresh), black peppercorns, mustard – Dijon & wholeseed, ground cumin, paprika, basil, cloves, coriander, tumeric, garlic paste, curry powder, curry pastes.
- **FRUITS** – best to choose those in season – all citrus fruits, cherries, plums, apples, bananas, pears, peaches, apricots, figs, nectarines, berries of all varieties, water melon, honeydew melon, grapes and custard apples

Toasting Seeds and Nuts

The easiest method for most seeds (such as sesame and caraway), and pine nuts is to pre-heat a frypan, add a small amount of oil, sprinkle the seeds or nuts in the pan and gently turn with a wooden spoon until lightly toasted. Watch them carefully as they can burn very quickly. Remove them from the frypan and place on absorbent paper to cool.

Coconut (shredded, flaked or fine) can be toasted in the same way as the seeds, or alternatively spread evenly on a tray and placed in a moderate oven until toasted. With either method, the coconut must be watched carefully as it will burn quickly.

Almonds and other nuts can be dry roasted over moderate heat in a pan, or on a tray in a moderate oven, or if you wish, use the same method as for the seeds.

If prepared in advance the toasted nuts or seeds can be stored in an airtight container in your pantry or kitchen cupboard. Remember to eat plenty of your nuts raw (un-roasted) as they are very healthy when raw.

Preparing Legumes

Legumes consist of beans, peas and lentils. Many varieties are now available in cans and only need to be rinsed and drained before being combined with other ingredients. Alternatively you can prepare them from the dried product with the following method -

Soak the legumes in a saucepan with two to three times their volume of cold water.

It is often most convenient to soak them overnight.

Drain the water, rinse the beans, and add new water using three times the amount of water as the beans. Bring the water to the boil and simmer the beans until they are tender. Avoid adding salt to the water. Drain the water off.

Cooking times will vary according to the size and type of the legume.

Legumes are cooked when they are just soft when you squeeze them.

Do not overcook, or the legumes will become "mushy" and are unsuitable for salads. If overcooked they can be used in soups or casseroles. You can freeze any left over legumes in an airtight freezer bag, draw as much air from the bag as you can, seal and freeze.

You can also store cooked beans in an airtight container for several days in the fridge.

The GI of cooked beans is generally lower than that of canned beans, however it is acceptable to use canned beans for convenience.

22

Chapter Twenty Two

Balancing the Food Groups

Balancing the Food Groups

The maintenance eating plan in this book is designed to provide an approximate total calorie breakdown as follows –

- 40 to 45% from low GI carbohydrates
- 25 to 30% from healthy fats with approximately 10% of the fat supplied being saturated.
- 25 to 30% from first class lean protein

These percentages are approximations and can be varied by around 10% without upsetting your metabolism. If you do decide that you want to eat a meal with a higher percentage of carbohydrate, it is very important to choose carbohydrates with a low Glycaemic Index – *see page 121*. If you feel that you desire to eat a meal with more fat, then choose the healthy fats from eggs, cold pressed oils, oily fish or any seafood, stir-fried vegetables, avocados and nuts. Avoid deep fried foods. If you feel you need more protein make sure that you choose only fresh and lean types of protein.

Lets look at a few examples to see how the theory works. If you are eating a total of 2,000 calories daily here is a possible breakdown of food groups –

Percentage	Calories	Food Group
100%	2000	all groups
40% C	800	200 grams carbohydrate (4 calories per gram)
30% F	600	67 grams fat (9 calories per gram)
30% P	600	150 grams protein (4 calories per gram)

Foot Note: Carbohydrates = C, Protein = P, Fat = F

As another example, if you are eating a total of 1200 calories daily here is a possible breakdown of food groups –

Percentage	Calories	Food Group
100%	1200	all groups
40% C	480	120 grams carbohydrate (4 cals per gram)
30% F	360	40 grams fat (9 cals per gram)
30% P	360	90 grams protein (4 cals per gram)

Foot Note: Carbohydrates = C, Protein = P, Fat = F

Metabolically Resistant People

There are some people who are extremely resistant to losing weight even though they have spent a life time dieting. They have often tried every possible diet including low-fat low-calorie diets with only a total calorie content of 600 calories per day. Many of them have given up in desperation after a lifetime of being a yoyo dieter. Many of these metabolically resistant people are overly sensitive to "normal" or conventionally accepted amounts of carbohydrate. They find that they are unable to lose weight **initially** with 40% of daily calories being provided by carbohydrate. **To enable weight loss to begin and kick-start the metabolism** in these difficult resistant patients, it is often necessary to reduce the percentage of daily calories provided by carbohydrate to much lower levels. Some popular high-protein high-fat diets allow as little as 6 to 18% of daily calories to be obtained from carbohydrate. There is no doubt that this dramatic strategy can work for these very resistant patients, and some times it can be very effective to reduce the dietary carbohydrate intake to these extremely low levels. This can allow weight loss to begin.

Lets take a look at 2 examples of this extremely low carbohydrate diet –

Let us say you are eating 1200 calories a day with only 10% of these calories being provided by carbohydrate foods

Percentage	Calories	Food Group
100%	1200	all groups
10% C	120	30 grams carbohydrate (4 cals per gram)
45% F	540	60 grams fat (9 cals per gram)
45% P	540	135 grams protein (4 cals per gram)

Foot Note: Carbohydrates = C, Protein = P, Fat = F

Let us say you are eating 1200 calories a day with only 6% of these calories being provided by carbohydrate foods

Percentage	Calories	Food Group
100%	1200	all groups
6% C	72	18 grams carbohydrate (4 calories per gram)
47% F	564	63 grams fat (9 calories per gram)
47% P	564	141 grams protein (4 calories per gram)

Foot Note: Carbohydrates = C, Protein = P, Fat = F

There are several diets like those on *page 239*, with extremely low amounts of carbohydrate, which are being followed by patients under the supervision of naturopaths and doctors. These diets will certainly put you into a state of ketosis and quick fat burning and can be very effective at **initialising weight loss** in metabolically resistant patients.

These extremely low carbohydrate diets can only be followed under supervision by a health care professional, and are not practical to accept as a way of life for long periods of time. You can see from the tables on *page 239,* that when the carbohydrate intake is drastically reduced, it is necessary to greatly increase the amount of fat and protein in the diet to meet calorie requirements. If these very large amounts of protein and/or fat are consumed for long periods, you will need to be closely supervised by your doctor. Otherwise you may find that metabolic problems such as high uric acid levels, high LDL cholesterol and constipation occur. When you are on these extremely low carbohydrate diets, you will need to eat large amounts of green leafy vegetables and salad greens to support your kidney and liver function and to avoid constipation. The use of the Ketostix urine testing strips can be helpful when you are trying to determine the maximum daily amount of carbohydrate that you can eat, before you bust out of the fat burning zone. You need to find the daily amount of carbohydrate that will keep the Ketostix testing in the purple colour range, which indicates that you are in the fat burning zone. While in the fat burning zone you will be eliminating enough ketones in the urine to make the Ketostix turn purple. If you eat too much carbohydrate your metabolism will shift out of the fat burning zone into the carbohydrate burning zone, and the excretion of ketones in the urine will fall to lower levels, that are insufficient to turn the Ketostix purple. Everyone has an individual metabolism, but generally less than 20gms of carbohydrate daily, will keep you well and truly in the fat burning and ketone-producing zone. Some people may find that they can eat more than 20gms of carbohydrate daily, and still stay in the fat burning zone with purple Ketostix. This takes some trial and error but eventually you will find the maximum daily intake of carbohydrate that allows you to stay in the fat burning zone of ketosis with purple Ketostix. You can use the carbohydrate counter on *page 123 - 130* to help you work this out.

Use of Ketostix urine testing strips

Amount of Ketones in urine	Colour Change
Negative (no ketones)	very light pink
Trace = 0.5mmol/L	light pink
Small = 1.5mmol/L	bright pink
Moderate = 4mmol/L	purple
Large = 8mmol/L	dark purple
Very large = 16mmol/L	very dark purple

There is a colour code on the Ketostix container to compare your testing strips with to determine the amount of ketones in your urine. The directions on the container must be followed exactly to get an accurate measurement. Ketostix testing strips can be purchased from your local pharmacy.

Extra points

Also remember it is not only how **much** you eat that's important, but rather **what** you eat that will cause the chemical and hormonal imbalances that lead to weight excess and Syndrome X. The real plague is refined carbohydrate, which will send your insulin levels sky rocketing. I well remember a well-known naturopath in Adelaide South Australia, who used to tell his patients that white sugar should be called "white death".

If you are hungry please eat enough to satisfy your own natural hunger. Your appetite will vary according to the amount of exercise you do, and also according to your body weight. So if you need food, eat healthy food choices from our Syndrome X Shopping List – *see page 230 - 234.*

Our recipes provide plenty of raw fruits and vegetables to provide anti-oxidants and cancer fighting phyto-nutrients. Raw foods are essential to improve your liver function and cleanse the lymphatic system, and some raw foods should be eaten with **EVERY** meal.

The meals largely composed of seafood, meat, poultry, eggs or legumes are higher in protein than meals based upon vegetables only. However remember that you can get first class protein by combining 3 of the following 4 groups at **one meal** –
Legumes - beans, peas and lentils.
Grains – rice, tapioca, arrowroot, maize, millet, buckwheat, sago, amaranth, wheat, rye, barley, oats, spelt, kamut, quinoa, teff and semolina.
Nuts of all varieties – almonds, cashews, peanuts, Brazil nuts, hazelnuts, pecans, walnuts, macadamia and pine nuts etc.
Seeds – sesame, sunflower, flaxseed, and pumpkin seeds.

23

Chapter Twenty Three

THE SYNDROME X DIET

The 12-Week Metabolic Weight Loss Eating Plan

The 12 - Week Metabolic Weight Loss Eating Plan

Stage One

The First Stage = 6 weeks of very low carbohydrate intake

- During these 6 weeks you can ***choose the recipes in this book that are marked with a "★"***, which are lower in carbohydrate and higher in protein.
- You will ***not*** be able to eat any of the following –
  Bread, pasta, rice, noodles, cakes, biscuits, crackers, muffins, lollies, chocolate, desserts or starchy vegetables (potatoes, pumpkin, parsnip, swede) during these 6 weeks.
- You will be more successful if you choose the low carbohydrate vegetables – *see page 123,* and the low carbohydrate green leafy salads, accompanied by pure protein such as eggs, seafood and lean fresh meat.
- You can have legumes but be aware that although they have a low GI, they contain significant amounts of carbohydrate. Thus you should eat legumes in moderation during this stage one.
- You can have 2 serves of fresh fruits daily, but avoid the fruits high in sugar such as bananas, mango, pears, pineapple and papaya.
- You will be more successful if you avoid milk of any kind in your tea and coffee.

During stage one, your rate of weight loss will vary, according to –

- The state of your liver
- The degree with which you suffer from Syndrome X.

Some people can expect a weekly weight loss of half to one kilogram (one to two pounds), while in others the rate of weight loss may be much more than this.

There will be some of you who will benefit by staying on stage one for longer than 6 weeks. This would apply if you have more than 20 kilograms (44 pounds) of weight to lose, or if you have a fatty liver. It would also apply if you have been a chronic yoyo dieter and/or have had Syndrome X for many years. Please be patient, as if you have a fatty liver, it can take 2 to 3 years to reverse this dangerous condition.

For those who want more rapid weight loss-

I suggest that you follow a very low carbohydrate diet (say less than 20 to 40grams of carbohydrate daily), under the close supervision of your health care professional.

If you want to get in touch with a suitable professional who has expertise in this area please call the Health Advisory Service on 02 4655 8855.

Stage Two

The Second stage = 6 weeks of low carbohydrate intake

- During these 6 weeks you are able to use **any of the recipes in this book**. However you should avoid the desserts.
- You will be allowed to have one slice of bread daily **and** one serving of starchy vegetables daily.
- You can have 2 to 3 serves of fresh fruit daily, but avoid papaya, pineapple, mangos and bananas.
- You can replace the one slice of bread with extra pasta, or a grain such as brown rice if desired.

Stage Three

Stage Three = Maintenance eating plan

- You can begin the maintenance program once you have reached your desired weight, or if you do not want to continue with stage two after 6 weeks.
- Stage three provides approximately 40 to 45% of daily calories from carbohydrate.
- You can use **any of the recipes in this book** and may have 2 to 3 desserts a week.
- You can have 2 to 3 serves of any fresh fruit daily.
- You are allowed to have 2 slices of bread daily and one serve of starchy vegetables daily, or 1 slice of bread **and** two serves of starchy vegetables daily.
- You can replace the 2 slices of bread with pasta or noodles, or more starchy vegetables or a grain such as brown rice if desired.

Extra Tips:

• Free foods

Salad vegetables and green vegetables are free foods, and you may eat as much of these as you like.

• For those who are short of time and money!

You may make any of your meals from canned seafood, eggs, lean fresh meats, protein powder, canned legumes, our high protein bean salad recipes *(see page 260 - 267)*, one to two slices of low carbohydrate bread, home made muesli *(see recipe page 255)*, and plenty of fresh salads and vegetables. If you are short of money, you may purchase the baking or loose nuts in the supermarkets, as these are generally cheaper.

Remember every time you eat protein, make sure you add some fibrous fruits or vegetables to prevent constipation.

Remember every time you eat carbohydrate, try to include some protein, as this will reduce the possible rise in blood sugar levels after eating.

Boil 6 eggs at a time, so they are ready in the fridge for you to have a snack.

• Spicy Foods can boost a sluggish metabolism

Many of the recipes in this book contain natural herbs, spicy vegetables and spices that are more commonly used in Asian cuisine.

Examples of these include –

Garlic, onion, chilli, curry, ginger, lime leaves, lemon grass, garam masala, tandoori paste, tamarind paste, coriander, dill, basil, mint, tumeric, cumin, cardamom, cinnamon, cloves, nutmeg, paprika, black pepper and others.

We have included these spices and herbs, as research has shown that spicy food and natural herbs are able to speed up the metabolic rate, which is useful for those who are metabolically resistant and do not burn fat easily. Furthermore these natural ingredients add wonderful new and often exotic flavours to the meals, and are excellent substitutes for sugar and processed sauces, which are often full of artificial preservatives and colourings.

So do not be surprised to find that you start to lose weight more easily when you include these natural herbs and spices in your meals. For those who do not like the taste or effect of spicy food, it is not a problem to exclude them, as the balance of the food groups in our recipes will still ensure that your metabolism is improved.

- **Acidic substances**

Acidic substances such as vinegar and lemon juice have a beneficial effect upon the metabolism. They may also help the digestive process when they are consumed with a meal. It has also been found that the acid content in tart tasting foods, such as vinegar and lemon, can help to moderate the blood sugar elevation that follows the ingestion of high GI carbohydrates. So it is good to include these things with a meal, and apple cider vinegar is the best vinegar of all to use regularly as part of a salad dressing. Those who suffer with poor digestion of food can slowly sip a small glass of water containing a dessertspoon of apple cider vinegar during a meal.

- **How much is one serving of carbohydrate?**

4 cracker biscuits
½ cup cooked pasta, cooked cereal, cooked rice
1 cup cooked legumes
1 cup raw muesli
1 slice of bread
2 sweet biscuits
2 cups raw leafy vegetables
1 cup cooked mixed vegetables
½ cup cooked potatoes
1 cup vegetable juice
1 piece fresh fruit
¼ cup dried fruit

You can interchange these servings.

24

Chapter Twenty Four

RECIPES

Healthy additions to meals

Linseed, Sunflower seeds and Almonds Mixture (LSA)

Much has been written about the benefits of linseed (flaxseed) in our diets, and we now find it in many of our bread and cereal products. Since the introduction of "LSA" - Linseed, Sunflower seed, and Almonds some time ago, many of us have added this mixture to our favourite recipes such as smoothie drinks, cereals, soups, dips, casseroles, cakes, biscuits, desserts, in fact anything which can include a meal substance. LSA is an excellent source of healthy essential fatty acids, calcium, phosphorus, potassium, iron, magnesium, copper, manganese, selenium, vitamin A, vitamin E and B group vitamins.

You can also use "LAA" - Linseed, Alfalfa seeds and Almonds. Alfalfa seeds will provide plant hormones, chlorophyll (a natural cleanser), and many of the essential vitamins and minerals.

★ LAA Recipe

4 tbsp Linseed (flaxseed)
1 tbsp Alfalfa seeds
3 tbsp Almonds
Use a coffee grinder or food processor, and grind to a fine meal.
Store in an airtight container in the refrigerator or freezer.
Use as required but re-seal to retain freshness. Use in recipes, in a similar way to LSA.

★ LSA Recipe

3 cups Linseed (flaxseed)
1 cup Almonds
2 cups Sunflower seeds
(For smaller quantities use tablespoons instead of cups)
Use a coffee grinder or food processor and grind to a fine meal.
Store in an airtight container in the refrigerator or freezer. Use as required but re-seal to retain freshness.
Start your day with LSA or LAA. Sprinkle it over your usual cereal, on sandwiches, whole meal toast, with tahini, or a small amount of nut paste (no butter or margarine).

If you enjoy fresh fruit for breakfast, chop up a banana, some melon, pears, apples, oranges, kiwi fruit, strawberries, or any of your preferred fruits, and sprinkle with LSA or LAA.

★ Gomasio

Gomasio is a Japanese condiment made from sesame seeds and salt. It is very high in calcium and other beneficial minerals. Gomasio adds a delicious flavour to any savoury meal. Try it instead of salt.

Ingredients:

1	part unrefined sea salt
23	parts hulled sesame seeds

Preparation:

Heat a heavy frying pan
Add sea salt and stir gently as it dries out
Add sesame seeds, combine with the salt
Stir continuously until the sesame seeds are golden brown, be careful not to burn them – they are ready when a seed can be crushed easily between your thumb and finger
Pour the mix into a grinding bowl
Grind the mixture, keep it quite coarse as it is nice to chew
Allow to cool before storing

A delicious variation of Gomasio is-

2 tbsp dry roasted sesame seeds (crushed), 2 tbsp water & 2tbsp tamari sauce. This is great with steamed vegetables, or over half an avocado filled with seafood.

★ SEA VEGETABLE CONDIMENT

Ingredients:

30g	dry arame
1tbsp	black vinegar
1/2tbsp	shoyu sauce
3	drops chilli oil
1/2tbsp	sesame oil
1/2	bunch chives, chopped into ½ cm lengths

Preparation:

Soak the arame in boiling water for 5 minutes
Drain well and set aside
Mix the vinegar, shoyu and chilli oil
Heat a frying pan, add the sesame oil
Sauté the chives for 1 minute
Add the arame and cook for another 2 minutes

Pour in the liquids
Simmer gently until most of the liquid has gone
Spoon into a small bowl and serve with your vegetables and/or grains.
Serves 6

★ TAHINI DRESSING

Ingredients:

4tbsp tahini
1 clove garlic, crushed
1tbsp lemon juice
1tbsp tamari
Cold water

Preparation:

Place all ingredients in a jar and mix well and shake, or mix in a blender
The tahini will make the dressing quite thick, so add cold water to make to your desired consistency

★ TOFU DRESSING

Ingredients:

200g fresh silken tofu, drained
2tbsp lemon juice
2tbsp cold pressed olive oil
1 tbsp tamari
1tsp red miso
4tbsp tahini
Add water to liquefy

Preparation:

Blend all ingredients until smooth
Serve on any hot vegetables, or as a salad dressing
Makes 1 cup

★ MOROCCAN PRESERVED LEMONS

Once you have allowed them to sit for 8 weeks, the preserved lemons can be added to many hot or cold dishes. They are delicious placed in rice during cooking, fabulous with chicken - while cooking or as a garnish, tasty with fish in any way. They are also great in vegetable stir-fries, thinly sliced and tossed in at the end of cooking. The Moroccan lemon oil is also delicious used in most recipes, especially Asian dishes, in place of other cooking oil. It is also nice as part of a salad dressing.

Ingredients

10	lemons, scrubbed and washed
2	cinnamon sticks
4	cardamom pods
1litre	cold pressed canola oil
1	large jar with air tight lid

Plenty of sea salt to cover the lemons

Preparation

Place the jar in a cold oven
Turn the oven on and turn up to 150C, leave for about 15 minutes, to sterilise the jar
Cut the lemons into quarters
Cover the fruit part of the lemons in a layer of salt
Layer the salted lemons into a ceramic bowl, be careful not to spill the salt
Cover them with a tea towel and leave for 24 hours
Pour out liquid and discard, be careful not to spill the salt
Place salted lemons into the sterilised glass jar with lid
Add cinnamon and cardamom pods
Pour canola oil over the top – until covered
Leave for 8 weeks in a cool dark place

★ Olive Tapenade

150g green or black pitted olives
4 anchovies (rinsed)
2 garlic cloves, peeled
2 tbsp capers
1 tbsp lemon juice
Freshly ground black pepper
Cold pressed olive oil
Place all ingredients in a blender
Dribble in olive oil into the mix while blending until it is of smooth and spreadable consistency

Audrey Tea's Natural Soy Mayonnaise

Mayonnaise Version One

Great with seafood cocktails and salads such as coleslaw

½ cup	soy mayonnaise
¼ cup	Balsamic or apple cider vinegar or lemon juice
2 tsp	tomato paste
½ tsp	horseradish sauce

1 tsp	minced garlic (optional)
¼ tsp	lemon pepper or black pepper and salt
Pinch	of chilli powder or 2 to 3 drops Tabasco sauce ***(optional)***

Shake all together in a screw top jar and refrigerate

Mayonnaise Version Two

½ cup	soy mayonnaise
1 tbsp	finely chopped gherkin
1 dsp	fresh chopped parsley
¼ tsp	lemon pepper or black pepper and salt
½ tsp	horseradish sauce

Shake all together in a screw top jar and refrigerate

Mayonnaise Version Three

½ cup	soy mayonnaise
¼ cup	apple cider vinegar or lemon juice
1 level tsp	dry mustard powder
½ tsp	ground oregano
½ tsp	lemon pepper or black pepper and salt

Shake all together in a screw top jar and refrigerate

if you prefer a sweeter mayonnaise substitute fresh orange juice for vinegar.

Audrey Tea's Handy Cooking Hints

- Be confident when you cook and don't be intimidated by a long list of ingredients.
- Try not to substitute any of the oils or soy products, because these are specially chosen for your health and well being.
- Herbs and seasonings can be used to individual taste and may be adjusted before serving.
- All frozen serves should be placed in the freezer as soon as possible. This is a very practical and economical way to save on cooking time, and yet have a quickly prepared tasty meal.
- Square and oblong containers are best for freezing as they pack better and save space. Remember to label and date each pack.

Now start preparing and good luck! I know that you will be rewarded for your time, when you taste these delicious, healthy and satisfying "liver friendly meals".

Note - These recipes are not designed for just one person, and they are suitable to serve to the whole family. However, if you live alone, you can halve the ingredient amounts, and freeze food left over for tomorrow.

BREAKFAST RECIPE CHOICES

MUESLI WITH THE LOT

2 cups rolled oats
2 cups processed bran
1 cup oat bran
1 cup rice bran
½ cup natural sultanas
½ cup currants
½ cup chopped dried apricots
½ cup chopped almonds
½ cup Pepitas (green pumpkin seeds)
½ cup Sunflower seeds

Mix all together - store in an airtight container

Breakfast is a very important start to your day. This muesli mix is a "***First Class Protein***", which is essential for those with Syndrome X to start the day.

1 Serve - 2 to 4 tablespoons muesli with soymilk, almond milk, and rice milk or oat milk or protein powder.

You may add some chunks of fresh fruit if desired.

You may add one dessertspoon LSA and one teaspoon lecithin if desired.

A large quantity of this muesli recipe can be made and stored in an airtight container and will keep well if you sticky tape some bay leaves on the inside of the lid.

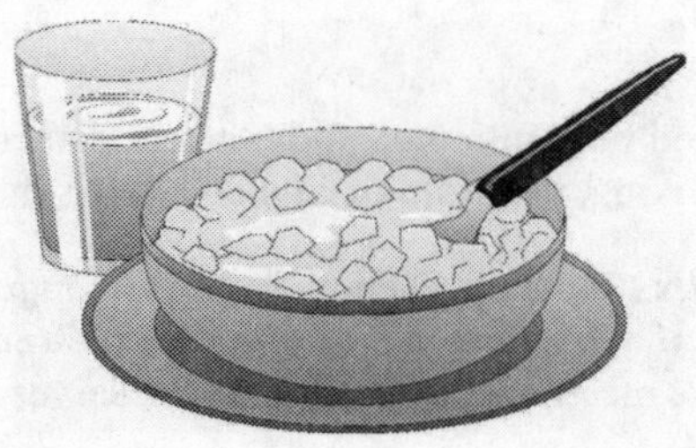

★ LOW CARBOHYDRATE MUESLI

2 cups rolled oats
2 cups processed bran (similar in texture to Kellogg's Allbran or Vogel's Soy & Linseed with no added sugar)
1 cup oat bran
1 cup rice bran
1 tbsp natural sultanas
2 tbsp chopped dried apricots
½ cup chopped almonds
½ cup pepitas (green pumpkin seeds)
½ cup sunflower seeds

Mix all together - store in an airtight container
This low carbohydrate muesli mix is a "***First Class Protein***", which is essential for those with Syndrome X to start the day.
1 Serve - 2 to 4 tablespoons muesli with soymilk, almond milk, and rice milk or oat milk or protein powder
You may add one dessertspoon L.S.A. and one teaspoon lecithin if desired.
A large quantity of this muesli recipe can be made and stored in an airtight container and will keep well if you sticky tape some bay leaves on the inside of the lid.

★ Omelette

Use any combination of vegetables and meat that you enjoy – such as chicken, avocado, salmon, tuna, tomato, broccoli finely chopped, spinach, onion, chives, garlic, chilli, black pepper, sea salt, coriander, sun-dried tomatoes (chopped) etc. Serves one person.

Method one

Combine 2 eggs in a bowl and whisk, add all the other chopped ingredients and mix, pour into fry pan on a low heat. Then flip mixture in the pan to cook the topside, or place pan under the grill to cook the top of the omelette.

Method two

Beat the 2 eggs and pour into pan, add other ingredients on top of one half of eggs as cooking, then fold other side of eggs over when cooked.

★ Poached eggs (2 to 3 eggs) cooked with asparagus and their juice. One slice of toast if allowed, depending upon which stage of the eating plan you are on. A mixed raw vegetable juice. Serves one person.

★ **Grilled lean lamb chops** (2 chops) – remove all the fat. Grill in the griller with one tomato (halved) and mushrooms. Add salad vegetables. Serves one person.

★ **Tinned sardines** in oil or brine, and 2 slices of eggplant with field mushrooms, grilled. One fresh tomato and/or a raw vegetable juice. One slice of toast if allowed, depending upon which stage of the eating plan you are on. Serves one person.

★ **"Smoothie"** drink with 1 cup unsweetened soy, rice, oat or almond milk, or water plus two tablespoons of Synd-X protein powder, and one raw egg (optional) and 6 strawberries (or other berries) mixed in a blender. One dessertspoon of ground flaxseed can be added to the smoothie. * Water will be best for those who wish to make this low carbohydrate. Serves one person.

★ **Scrambled eggs** (2 to 3 eggs) made with soy or oat milk, seasoned with fresh herbs, pepper and salt. One slice of toast if allowed, depending upon which stage of the eating plan you are on. One piece fresh fruit or a mixed raw vegetable juice. Serves one person.

★ **Scrambled eggs** (2 to 3 eggs) cooked with thinly sliced mushrooms and chopped chives. One slice of toast if allowed, depending upon which stage of the eating plan you are on. One grapefruit. Serves one person.

"Bubble and Squeak" - Leftover mashed vegetables mixed together with 1 beaten egg and seasoning, rounded into patties and warmed through in a non-stick frypan. Serve with your favourite non-sweetened relish. One piece fresh fruit or a mixed raw vegetable juice. Serves one person.

Toast - one to two slices of wholegrain or sourdough bread, toasted and spread with tahini, and sprinkled with LSA. One piece fresh fruit or a mixed raw vegetable juice. Serves one person.

Baked beans (canned) warmed through with some chopped onion, tomato and capsicum and a sprinkle of chopped parsley. Sprinkle with one dessertspoon of LSA or LAA. One grapefruit. Serves one person.

Fruit breakfast - 1 slice cantaloupe, 1 orange, 1 pear. Chop fruit into bite size pieces. Serve with a large dollop of unsweetened soy yoghurt mixed with 1 to 2 tablespoons of Synd-X protein powder. Serves one person.

★ **Avocado and Salmon** – half large avocado peeled and chopped, 1/2 slice of pineapple, ¼ cup chopped almonds or any other chopped fresh nuts. Chop fruit, toss with nuts and sprinkle with 1 tablespoon chopped mint. Gently fold in the contents of a 110gm tin of pink salmon in brine (or tuna in brine). Serves one person.

Quick breakfast for those in a hurry -1 cup unsweetened soy, almond, rice or oat milk, 1 banana (or ½ cup berries or strawberries for less carbohydrate), 2 tablespoons of Synd-X protein powder, a dash of vanilla essence. Process all in blender until smooth, sprinkle with a little cinnamon. Serves one person.

★ **To make this quick breakfast low in carbohydrate**, use water instead of milk, and use 2 to 3 tablespoons of the Synd-X protein powder with the berries or strawberries instead of the banana. Serves one person.

★ **Hard-boiled eggs** chopped, (2 or 3 eggs), ¼ cup grated carrot, ½ cup chopped mixed fresh herbs (parsley, oregano & mint is a good mix). Toss together with a little cracked black pepper and 1 teaspoon chilli sauce (sweetened with a pinch of stevia powder and not containing added sugar). 2 to 3 olives on the side with a handful of alfalfa sprouts.One or two slices of wholemeal toast if allowed, depending upon which stage of the eating plan you are on. Serves one person.

★ **Fillet fresh fish** (1 large fillet) cooked in a non-stick frypan with a good squeeze of lemon juice and black pepper, to taste. A little chopped dill gives this a lovely flavour. Serve with 2 sticks of celery, half a vine ripened tomato and a handful of alfalfa or bean sprouts, or a mixed raw vegetable juice. Serves one person.

★ **Soybeans** (fresh or canned) – ½ cup, cooked until tender and drained. Return beans to the saucepan and add 1 chopped tomato (can use tinned if more convenient), 1 chopped boiled egg, I to 2 tbsp chives, 1 large clove garlic minced (can use prepared from a jar) or chopped red onion. Warm through, season with salt and pepper. The soybeans can be replaced with tofu if preferred. Serve with handful of alfalfa or bean sprouts. Serves one person.

Cooked fruit - 1 cupful of cooked chopped apple, pear and any stone fruit, (without added sugar), sprinkle over with 1-tsp ground flaxseed,

1-tbsp of Synd-X protein powder and 1-tbsp of chopped/ground almonds. Can add a pinch of stevia powder if desired to sweeten. Serves one person.

★ **Herrings or kippers** – tinned, either in brine or oil, topped with chopped spring onions and chopped parsley or coriander, and a generous squeeze of lemon juice. Can serve hot or cold with 3 to 4 olives, and a handful of bean sprouts. One grapefruit. Serves one person.

★ **Lean steak** - grilled or pan-cooked, with 1 egg poached in non-stick pan, served with half grilled tomato, chopped chives and celery, black pepper and sea salt, minced chilli or minced garlic (optional). One grapefruit. Serves one person.

Energising drinks to accompany breakfast meals

A mixed vegetable juice of your choice, or a smoothie of your choice. Remember you are allowed only 2 to 3 pieces of fruit a day, so watch that you don't use your daily allowance at one time. Those on stage one of the eating plan can only have 2 serves of fresh fruit daily. Strawberries, apricots, honeydew melon, green grapes, berries, cherries and prunes are the lower carbohydrate fruits to choose if possible.Some beverage suggestions are:

★ Tomato Refresher and Vitamin C booster

Juice enough raw tomato and green apple (2/3 tomato and 1/3 apple mixture) to make about 250 mls to 300 mls or 1 large cup. Also juice ½ to 1 clove garlic (optional), 2 to 3 fresh basil leaves, and 4 fresh mint leaves. For extra spice add 2-3 drops of Tabasco sauce. Have this with a 125gm tin of sardines in oil, or a 125gm tin of tuna flavoured with herbs or chilli. One slice of wholemeal or sourdough bread with olive oil and sliced tomatoes, depending upon which stage of the eating plan you are on.

Melon Pep to start your day

2 slices watermelon – leave some of the inner skin on melon, 2 thick stems of celery and tops, 4-6 mint or sage leaves. Process all in juicer. Serve with 1 lean grilled chop, a small piece of grilled steak or fish, or 2 eggs cooked any way except fried.

Tropical breakfast drink

1 cup coconut milk (canned is acceptable)
1 peach or similar stone fruit
3 - 4 strawberries

1 raw egg or 2 Tbsp of Synd-X protein powder
Trim fruit and place all ingredients in blender and process until silky smooth. Sprinkle with dried coconut and ground almonds to serve.

Breakfast notes
Vegetables are ideally eaten with every meal, either fresh as a salad, or cooked, as in leftovers from the night before. The vegetables may be replaced with 1 to 2 pieces of raw fruit at breakfast or lunchtime. Keep it as simple as possible for breakfast as this is usually a very busy time of the day.

If you have a suitable salad left over from the previous evening then use that. It will remain fresh overnight if you store it in an airtight bowl or covered with gladwrap. Otherwise prepare strips, chunks or bite size pieces of salad, ie, celery, snow peas, carrots, capsicum, cauliflower and broccoli florets, bean sprouts, any type of lettuce, green beans, baby spinach leaves, watercress, spring onions or radish. Trim, wash and cut as desired and do enough to take for your lunch in an airtight plastic container.

SALADS

While offering you some tasty salad ideas, we are also trying to encourage you to sometimes just have a salad for a meal. This is very good for the liver and will promote weight loss.

To make the most of this idea, we are combining as many of the food groups as possible in our salads to create a "First Class Protein Salad" We are achieving this by including ingredients from at least three of the four food groups of Grains, Nuts, Seeds and Legumes (beans, peas and lentils) in one salad.

Any of the salads can be served with lean fresh cooked meat (or cold serves of this), poultry, eggs or seafood, but sometimes it is more convenient (especially for a workday lunch) to eat just a bowl of salad, and know that you are still eating a complete protein meal.

We are also including salads that can be prepared well ahead of time, and that will stay fresh for several days, if stored in an airtight container in the fridge.

Planning ahead always makes meal times a lot easier.

SALADS THAT WILL STORE COVERED BY GLADWRAP, OR IN AN AIRTIGHT CONTAINER IN THE FRIDGE, FOR A FEW DAYS PRIOR TO USE

Special Tabouli Salad

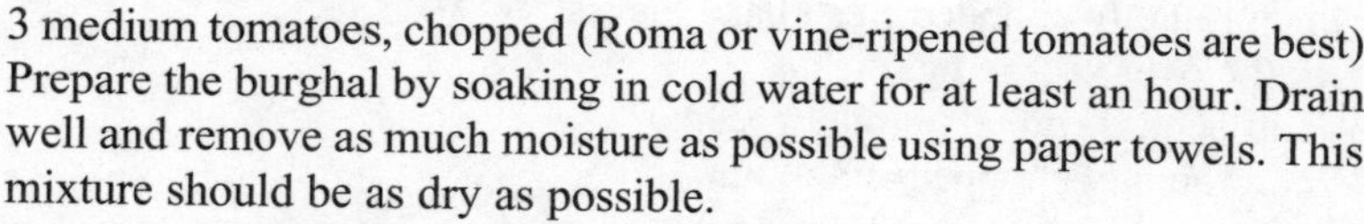

½ cup burghal (cracked wheat)
½ cup sunflower seeds
½ cup blanched almonds
1 tbsp sesame seeds
1 medium red onion chopped
4 cups chopped fresh parsley
4 cups chopped fresh mint leaves
¼ cup fresh lemon juice
¼ cup cold pressed olive oil
3 medium tomatoes, chopped (Roma or vine-ripened tomatoes are best)

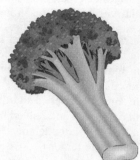

Prepare the burghal by soaking in cold water for at least an hour. Drain well and remove as much moisture as possible using paper towels. This mixture should be as dry as possible.

Toss all ingredients together, except the lemon juice and oil, and refrigerate. Place oil and lemon juice in a bottle or jar, season with salt and pepper to suit your own taste, shake well and toss through salad just prior to serving. Serves 4 to 6.

This salad can be eaten on its own as a meal, as it contains 3 of the essential vegetarian food groups to provide a first class protein.

Spectacular Rice Salad

4 cups warm, rinsed and drained cooked brown rice
¼ cup of sultanas
½ cup each of chopped spring onions, chopped and de-seeded red capsicum, raw cashews or blanched almonds.
½ cup each of sunflower seeds and pepitas (green pumpkin seeds)

Mix together all the above ingredients in a salad bowl

To prepare the dressing in a screw top jar, shake together -

½ cup cold pressed olive oil
1/3 cup apple cider vinegar
1/3 cup soy sauce
1 to 2 cloves of crushed garlic, or 1 to 2 teaspoons of minced garlic from a jar
1 dessertspoon of commercially prepared curry powder, or your own recipe for curry powder, if preferred
½ teaspoon lemon pepper, or cracked black pepper & rock salt

Mix in the dressing while the rice mixture is still warm

Store in the fridge in a sealed container

This rice salad will keep for several days in an airtight container in the fridge. It can be eaten on its own as a meal, as it contains 3 of the essential vegetarian food groups to provide a first class protein, ie. a grain, a seed and a nut. Serves 4 to 6.

Sun-dried tomatoes and bean salad

400gm soybeans, (cooked or canned), drained and rinsed
400gm butter beans (or any white beans, cooked or canned), drained and rinsed
200gm roughly chopped sun-dried tomatoes in oil
200gm de-seeded and halved black olives
grated rind of 1 large lemon
juice of 1 large lemon
½ teaspoon cracked black pepper, or lemon pepper
½ cup roughly chopped fresh basil leaves
1 or 2 cloves crushed garlic
½ cup pepitas (green pumpkin seeds)
½ cup roughly chopped Brazil nuts
1 tablespoon cold pressed olive oil

Whisk together the oil, lemon juice, pepper and garlic
In another large bowl combine all of the other ingredients
Pour on oil and lemon juice mixture and toss gently

Can be served on whole lettuce leaves as a complete meal, or as a side salad for fish and poultry. Serves 6.

This bean salad will keep for several days in an airtight container in the fridge. It can be eaten on its own as a meal, as it contains 3 of the essential vegetarian food groups to provide a first class protein.

It is an ideal salad to use as a workplace lunch.

★ Zesty Beetroot, Mushroom and Cucumber Salad

300gm Lebanese cucumber, finely chopped or sliced into small julienne pieces
1 large raw beetroot, peeled and finely chopped or sliced into small julienne pieces
½ avocado, chopped
1 medium red onion, finely chopped
1 cup mushrooms, washed and chopped
2 tablespoons fresh mint leaves, finely chopped
1 teaspoon grated lemon rind
1/3 cup lemon juice
1 teaspoon coarse cooking salt or sea salt

Place cucumber in a colander
Sprinkle the salt over the cucumber and allow to stand for 15mins
Rinse and drain the cucumber, and remove as much moisture as possible with absorbent paper
Combine all of the remaining ingredients together and toss with the cucumber
This salad is ideal to serve with warm cooked lamb or beef, or as a side dish for grilled fish. Will store in fridge for 2 days. Serves 4 to 6.

Mixed Bean Salad

1 can of 3 or 4-bean mix, or any beans of your choice – remember that soybeans are low in carbohydrate and have a low Glycaemic Index.
1 Lebanese cucumber, washed and diced
1 medium red onion, sliced
1 large tomato, de-seeded and diced
1 capsicum, de-seeded and cut into fine strips
2 sticks celery, chopped
1/3 cup fresh parsley, chopped
1 cup brown rice, cooked (optional)
½ cup roasted unsalted peanuts

Dressing

¼ cup balsamic vinegar, or apple cider vinegar
¼ cup cold pressed olive oil
1 dessertspoon soy sauce
Drain and rinse the beans. Mix and combine the rice, vegetables and peanuts.
Shake dressing ingredients together, and gently fold into the salad mixture.
This bean salad is ideal to serve with hot or cold meat or fish, or as a very filling protein meal served on its own with lettuce and carrot sticks. Will store in fridge for 2-3 days. Serves 4 to 6.

The following salads are best made just prior to serving.

★ Hot and Spicy Salad with Cool Cucumber Dressing

1 cup red skinned radishes, thinly sliced
½ cup turnip, grated
1 cup red or green capsicum, thinly sliced
1 red onion, thinly sliced
1 cup celery, thinly sliced
1 or 2 small red chillies, de-seeded and thinly sliced (optional)

Cucumber dressing for Hot and Spicy Salad.

1 Lebanese cucumber (approx 200gm), chopped
200ml unsweetened soy yoghurt
½ cup fresh mint leaves, chopped
1 tablespoon fresh lemon juice
Process all of the dressing ingredients in a blender until smooth.
Combine all salad ingredients in a bowl and drizzle dressing through the salad mixture until combined.

Taste tip: This cucumber dressing is also suitable to use as a side condiment for hot and spicy curries, and is delicious with Cajun dishes. Serve with a few cucumber and celery sticks and dip them in the dressing. Serves 4 to 6.

Spinach Salad

125gm-baby spinach leaves, with stems trimmed off
400gm tin chick peas – rinsed and drained
1 small red capsicum, de-seeded and thinly sliced
½ medium red onion, thinly sliced
¼ cup pepitas (green pumpkin seeds)
½ cup raw hazelnuts or macadamia nuts

Dressing

¼ cup balsamic vinegar or apple cider vinegar
2 tablespoons cold pressed olive oil
1 teaspoon seedy mustard
1 clove crushed garlic
pinch of lemon pepper or cracked black pepper
salt to taste
Place all salad ingredients in a bowl and toss together
Place all dressing ingredients in a screw top jar and shake until well mixed
Pour dressing over salad just before serving.. Serves 4 to 6.

★ Cabbage Cucumber and Mint Salad

400gm green cucumber – Lebanese variety ideal
1 tsp coarse salt or sea salt
½ small cabbage, chopped finely (Chinese or savoy ideal)
3 tablespoons fresh mint leaves, chopped
1 tbsp sesame seeds toasted
½ cup walnuts

Dressing

1 teaspoon finely grated lemon rind

½ cup fresh lemon juice
1 teaspoon honey (or pinch of stevia powder)
1 teaspoon garlic, crushed or minced
Slice, or thinly julienne cucumber, sprinkle with salt, and allow to stand for 15 mins
Rinse cucumber and pat dry with absorbent paper
Mix salad ingredients together
Place all dressing ingredients in a screw top jar, and shake until well mixed
Pour dressing over salad ¼ hour before serving and refrigerate until ready to serve.
Serve with Fish or BBQ meats. Serves 6.

★ Liver Cleansing Salad

1 cup broccoli florets
1 cup celery - diced
1 cup green capsicum - diced
1 cup green beans - chopped
4 to 6 spring onions - tops and all chopped
½ cup snow peas - trimmed
1 cup parsley - chopped
1 cup cucumber , Lebanese or small continental
A few red cherry tomatoes to garnish

Dressing

1 cup cold pressed sesame oil or olive oil
1 tablespoon fresh garlic – crushed (optional)
½ cup fresh squeezed lemon juice
½ teaspoon dried cumin
½ teaspoon lemon pepper or cracked black pepper & sea salt
Put all ingredients into a jar, with the lid on shake until well mixed.

Preparation:

Blanch broccoli in boiling water for 1 minute, drain, run under cold water and drain again.
Score cucumber skin with a fork and rinse under cold water and dice.
Toss all ingredients together.
Serves 6 - 8
You can halve the ingredients for a small salad. This salad will last 1 to 2 days.
If you still have some left over, toss it in a pan with a little shredded cabbage for a stir-fry, or add it to a casserole.
A very tasty, versatile and no waste salad.

★ Nice and Spicy Salad

1 cup mung bean sprouts
1 cucumber, thinly sliced
½ cup chopped spring onions
1 medium red onion, thinly sliced
1 medium red capsicum, de-seeded and thinly sliced,
¼ cup fresh coriander, chopped
200gm cubed firm tofu
2 small red chillies, de-seeded and finely sliced (optional)
¾ cup raw or roasted peanuts or Brazil nuts or almonds, chopped
1 tablespoon toasted sesame seeds

Dressing

1 tablespoons hot chilli sauce (can sweeten with a pinch of stevia powder if desired)
2 tablespoons soy sauce
2 cups cold pressed olive oil
2 cups tomato paste
2 teaspoons fish sauce
2 teaspoons honey
¼ teaspoon ground ginger powder
Combine all salad ingredients
Combine all dressing ingredients in a screw top jar, shake until mixed well, then drizzle over salad before serving
This salad dressing is also very tasty when added to some hot cooked noodles as a meal. Serves 6.

★ Very Low Carbohydrate Salad

cup lettuce, torn
½ cup spinach leaves, chopped
½ cup cucumber, sliced
½ cup celery, sliced
½ cup mushrooms, sliced
tbsp bean sprouts
½ tomato
radishes, chopped
2 spring onions, sliced
Mix salad ingredients and toss in dressing made with cold pressed oil (flaxseed or olive), 1 tbsp hummus and juice of half a lemon
Serve with canned fish or boiled eggs. Serves 4 to 6.

★ Spinach and Avocado Salad

2 cups raw spinach, chopped
1 clove garlic, chopped (optional)
3tbsp spring onions, sliced

2 -hard boiled eggs, quartered
1 small tomato, chopped
½ avocado, chopped

Dressing

2 tsp fresh lemon juice
2 tbsp olive oil cold pressed
Mix ingredients in a bowl and drizzle over dressing. Serves 4 to 6.

★ Chef's Salad

1 cup washed lettuce leaves, torn
½ cup canned chickpeas
½ cup button mushrooms, chopped
½ cup celery, chopped
1 small tomato, chopped
30g turkey breast, sliced
1 boiled egg, quartered
Combine ingredients, and toss in dressing of choice. Serves 4 to 6.

Fruit and Nut Salad

1 red apple diced, skin on, core out
1 green apple diced, skin on, core out

1 cup	celery, diced
1	avocado diced
1	red onion in thin half rings
425g/15oz	unsweetened pineapple pieces (retain juice), or fresh pineapple
1 cup	parsley, chopped
1 cup	pecans or walnuts, chopped

Gently toss apples and avocado in pineapple juice, drain
Mix with all other ingredients. Serves 6 - 8

LUNCHES

Bean Salad

One 410g can 3 bean mix combination or any canned legumes of your choice.
½ red onion, thinly sliced
1 capsicum, seeded & thinly sliced
½ cup mint, chopped
½ cup pumpkin seeds
½ cup of pine nuts or chopped almonds
A good squeeze of lemon juice
Make enough for 2-3 serves as this will keep in airtight container for a couple of days. Serve with lettuce. Drizzle over some cold pressed olive or flaxseed oil if desired.

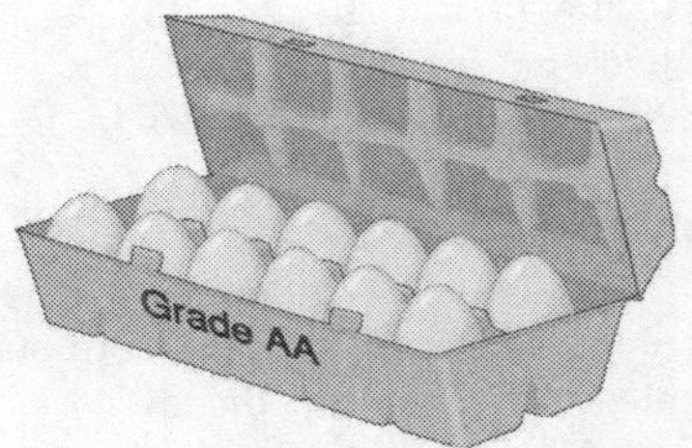

Salmon and Avocado

210g can pink salmon
½ avocado, chopped
1 onion, sliced
½ small cucumber, sliced
½ cup mushrooms, chopped
1 tomato, sliced
Season with black pepper and salt and a splash of balsamic vinegar or squeeze of fresh lemon. Don't discard bones from salmon – mash them into the fish. Can toss all ingredients together or arrange on plate. Serves 1 to 2.

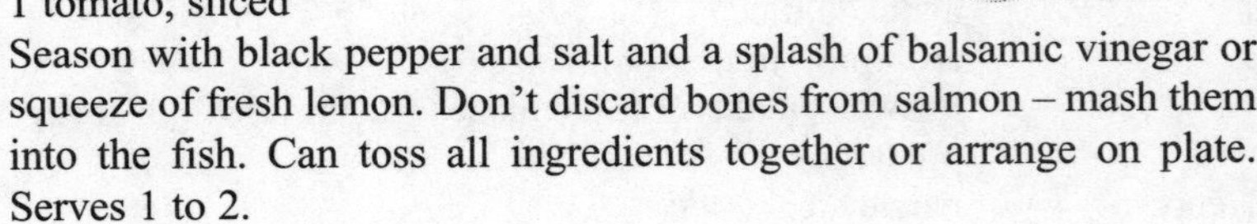

Zucchini slice

5 x 61 gr. Eggs, lightly beaten
400 gr. Zucchini, coarsely grated
2 medium carrots, coarsely grated
1 large onion, finely chopped
½ cup cold pressed olive oil
½ cup parsley, chopped
½ teaspoon lemon pepper or black pepper & sea salt
1 cup wholemeal SR flour
100 gr. soft tofu
1 tablespoon LSA
Combine all ingredients, except the flour, until well mixed and then fold in flour until well blended.
Pour into an oiled lamington tin 28 x 18 cm and bake in a moderate

oven for 30 to 40 minutes.

Serve warm with a fresh green salad. This slice can also be cut into wedges, and served cold for a picnic as finger food. Make enough to have some leftovers for another meal. Wrap and store in fridge. Serve with plenty of coleslaw and some grated fresh beetroot sprinkled with lemon juice. Serves 6 to 8.

★ Cold Roast Meat lunch

125g (4 oz) cold roast meat left over from a roast dinner, sliced
1 medium carrot, grated
1 capsicum, sliced
2 sticks of celery, sliced
1 tomato, sliced

Mix salad ingredients and toss a few chopped almonds into the salad. Drizzle with cold pressed olive oil and freshly squeezed lemon juice. Serves 1 to 2.

★ Hard boiled eggs

2 hard-boiled cold eggs, cut into quarters
1 cup lettuce, torn
½ cucumber, sliced
½ capsicum, sliced.

Serve with wedges of tomato and a handful of alfalfa or bean sprouts. Drizzle over cold pressed olive oil and apple cider vinegar. One slice of wholemeal or pumpernickel bread, depending upon which stage of the eating plan you are on. Serves 1.

Tasty Chunky Tomato Lentil Soup

One 810 gr. can of tomatoes, chopped
1 cup red lentils, soaked for one hour in 2 cups of boiling water
1 cup celery, chopped
1 tablespoon garlic, chopped
1 tablespoon fresh basil leaves, chopped
Garlic and basil according to your personal taste
½ cup parsley, chopped
1 large onion, chopped
½ teaspoon lemon pepper or cracked black pepper (optional)
½ teaspoon rock salt
2 tablespoon or more tomato paste
1 dessertspoon cold pressed olive oil

Preparation:

Brown onion and garlic in oil in a non-stick pan then add to all other ingredients in large pan. Simmer gently until all is tender for approx. one hour.

Add more water if necessary.

Season to taste before serving

This soup can be served chunky, or if preferred smooth - purée with a hand held food processor. Serve sprinkled with chopped parsley. Serves 6.

Suitable to freeze in meal size portions

Serve tomato and lentil soup, with a tossed salad (sprinkle chopped nuts and sesame seeds through the tossed salad)

★ Lamb loin chops with Salad

Grill 2 to 3 chops after removing the fat

1 cup assorted bean sprouts, washed

½ cup mushrooms, chopped

½ small cucumber, sliced

1 tomato, sliced

1 red capsicum, sliced

Toss salad ingredients together

Drizzle salad with fresh lemon juice or apple cider vinegar and cold pressed olive oil. Serves 1 to 2.

★ Grilled steak - (lean and fresh)

Serve with a large tossed salad with a large variety of raw vegetables, eg, green leaves of your choice, bean sprouts, thinly sliced salad onion, tomato and capsicum.

★ Shrimp (or crabmeat) and avocado with spicy dressing

1 cup lettuce leaves, torn into bite size pieces

210g of canned or fresh shrimps or crabmeat, drained

½ avocado, chopped

1 small Lebanese cucumber, diced

2-3 spring onions, chopped

1 red capsicum, chopped

½ cup alfalfa sprouts, washed

Toss all together and pour over dressing.

Dressing

You can have a simple dressing of cold pressed olive oil and freshly squeezed lemon juice, or an elaborate dressing consisting of-

½ avocado

¼ cup soy mayonnaise
1 teaspoon seeded mustard
1 dessertspoon cold pressed oil
1 dessertspoon lemon juice
1 dessertspoon tomato paste
1 teaspoon horseradish sauce
Blend all together in food processor. Store dressing in fridge in a screw top jar for up to 4 days. Serves 2.

★ Tomato and Basil Salad with Chilli Soy Dressing

4 Roma (egg shaped) or vine-ripened tomatoes, cut into quarters
1 red capsicum, de-seeded and thinly sliced
1 medium red onion, thinly sliced
2 sticks celery, sliced
¼ cup peanuts
6 fresh basil leaves, chopped.
Toss all together.

Dressing

1 tbsp chilli sauce (can sweeten with a pinch of stevia powder)
2 tbsp soy sauce
2 tbsp cold pressed sesame seed oil (or flaxseed oil)
1 tbsp tomato paste
2-3 cloves garlic crushed
2 tsp fish sauce
¼ - ½ tsp lemon pepper or cracked black pepper and sea salt
Combine all ingredients in a screw top jar and shake well. Pour over salad just before serving. Store remainder in fridge. Serves 2 to 3.

★ Sardine spread for Ryvita crackers

1 can sardines in oil, brine or tomato
1 clove garlic, crushed (optional)
10 black olives, pitted
1/2 cup parsley, chopped
1 tbsp apple cider vinegar
1 tbsp cold pressed olive oil
place all ingredients in food processor until combined
spread onto 2 or 3 Ryvita crackers
serve with celery and carrot sticks. Serves 1.

★ Tuna Vegetable Combo

1 220g can tuna or salmon
1 clove garlic, crushed

2 tbsp parsley, chopped
1 tbsp fresh basil, chopped
1 tbsp cold pressed olive oil
½ cup each of steamed zucchini, broccoli, leeks and mushrooms
Mix all ingredients in a large serving dish, toss and serve for 2.

★ Tuna and vegetable sticks with cucumber dip

One 125gm can of tuna or salmon, drained
1 Lebanese cucumber, grated
1/2 cup natural unsweetened soy yoghurt
2 tbsp fresh mint, chopped
1-2 cloves garlic crushed, or 1 tbsp chopped fresh chives
Plenty of raw vegetable sticks, ie, celery, carrot, cucumber or capsicum.
Combine cucumber with all the other ingredients and mix well. You may add salt and pepper or lemon pepper to your taste. Dip vegetable sticks into dip and enjoy. Refrigerate any leftovers for later. Serves 1 to 2.

★ Boiled egg and avocado with mustard dressing.

2 hard boiled eggs, chopped
½ cup bean sprouts or alfalfa sprouts, washed
1/2 avocado, chopped
2 sticks celery, chopped

Dressing

1 egg yolk, 2 tsp seedy mustard, 1 tbsp orange or lemon juice, 1 tbsp apple cider vinegar.
Place all ingredients in blender and process until smooth. Finally add ½ cup cold pressed olive oil, just letting it drizzle in while blender is still going. Taste and add a little lemon pepper or cracked black pepper if desired. Dressing will keep in fridge in screw top jar for a few days. To serve, pour dressing over sliced avocado with bean sprouts and celery sticks on the side. Serves 2.

★ Uncooked stuffed tomatoes

2 or more large tomatoes, vine ripened are great
100gm cooked crab meat or shrimps (canned is ok if unable to get fresh), drain
¼ cup carrot, grated
2 tbsp fresh peas or finely chopped canned asparagus
6 or more black olives, pitted and finely chopped
1 tbsp coriander, chopped
1 tbsp fresh basil leaves, chopped
Cut a small lid from tomatoes and gently scoop out flesh and seeds.

Mix all other ingredients together and spoon into tomato shells.

Dressing

Flesh & seeds from tomatoes
¼ cup cold pressed olive oil or flaxseed oil
pinch of white stevia powder or brown sugar
1 tbsp fresh dill, chopped
ground black pepper to taste

Blend flesh and seeds from tomatoes until smooth, fold in other ingredients. Pour into stuffed tomatoes, and drizzle remainder over a generous serve of mixed lettuce leaves and any other green salad vegetables that you fancy. Serves 2.

★ Paprika Chicken Drumsticks

8 chicken drumsticks, trimmed of skin and fat
1 tbsp wholegrain mustard
1 to 2 tsp paprika
3 tbsp cold pressed olive oil

Combine all ingredients in a bowl and add drumsticks. Turn drumsticks until well oiled.

Chicken can be barbecued or grilled, or place in oven covered in foil for 45 mins. Remove foil for last 15 minutes. Serve with strips of red and green capsicum, cooked broccoli and large green salad. These freeze well, so double the recipe if you like. Serves 4.

Jacket potatoes with bean filling

2 large potatoes boiled or baked in jacket until tender

Filling

One 210g can baked beans, or soybeans
½ medium onion, thinly sliced
½ capsicum, de-seeded and finely chopped
good pinch of chilli powder (optional)
2 tsp lemon pepper or cracked black pepper & sea salt
1 tbsp LSA

Put all ingredients, except potatoes, into a saucepan, mix and gently heat through. Cut a cross in top of each potato and squeeze to open. Spoon bean mixture into and over potatoes. You can replace the beans with cooked lean beef or lamb mince if desired. Pour over a little spicy plum or BBQ sauce and serve with a generous serve of coleslaw salad. Serves 2.

★ Cold Roast Meat with Mesclun salad

Slice desired amount of leftover cold roast meat and remove all fat. Place meat on a serving plate and serve with mesclun salad.

Mesclun is often found in about 250-gram packages, otherwise you will find it loose to choose the amount you need. The mesclun mixture should contain several varieties of lettuce, baby beetroot, spinach and silver beet leaves, watercress, flat parsley leaves and a sprinkle of edible flowers such as marigold or nasturtiums. Wash salad leaves, spin or pat dry.

Dressing – will cover about 250g mesclun

½ cup cold pressed flaxseed or olive oil
¼ cup apple cider vinegar
¼ cup lemon juice
¼ cup flat leaf parsley, very finely chopped
2 tsp dijon mustard

Shake together in a screw top jar and store in fridge. Serves 4.

★ Salmon with Tomato, Onion and Cucumber Salad

One 210gm can of salmon or tuna, drained
4 Roma (egg-shaped) or vine-ripened tomatoes, quartered or sliced
1 medium red onion, finely sliced
2 medium Lebanese cucumbers, halved and cut into chunks
2 tbsp fresh basil leaves, chopped
¼ tsp lemon pepper or cracked black pepper & sea salt
1 pinch sugar or white stevia powder
tsp balsamic vinegar
1 tbsp cold pressed olive oil

In a flat salad bowl layer the salad ingredients, sprinkling with seasoning as you layer them. Drizzle oil and vinegar over top, gently shake bowl, cover and stand in fridge for at least half an hour. Serve with salmon or tuna – eat enough to satisfy your hunger. This salad will store in fridge for 2 days. Serves 1 to 2.

★ Boiled eggs and snow pea salad

2 eggs – hard boiled - shell and cool.

Salad

250g green beans (or ½ green and ½ butter beans), washed
250g snow peas, washed
1 medium red onion, thinly sliced or chopped
¼ cup sunflower seeds
¼ cup shelled pumpkin seeds

Cut beans and snow peas into 5 cm pieces. Blanch beans and snow peas in boiling water for 1 minute. Rinse immediately under cold water and drain. Mix with all other ingredients.

Dressing

1-2 cloves garlic, crushed or minced
1 tbsp French mustard
2 tbsp freshly squeezed lemon juice
1/3 cup cold pressed oil
2 tbsp parsley, chopped

Whisk all dressing ingredients together in a bowl, pour over salad and toss gently. Serve with eggs. Serves 2.

★ Canned Fish served with Special Tabouli Salad

1 can sardines, herrings or kippers – in brine, oil or tomato sauce – mash the bones, do not discard them. (fish serves 2)

Salad (salad serves 6)

3 medium tomatoes, de-seeded and chopped
1/3 cup sunflower seeds
2 tbsp burghul, soaked in water for half an hour, drain & pat dry
1 medium red onion, chopped finely
4 cups fresh parsley leaves, chopped
2 cups fresh mint leaves, chopped

Dressing

¼ cup fresh lemon juice
¼ cup cold pressed olive oil

While the burghul is soaking, prepare all other ingredients and then toss all ingredients together until well mixed. Store covered in fridge. Will keep for 2-3 days. Serve with dressing.

★ Sliced chicken breast with salad

One chicken breast - remove skin from chicken – served hot or cold
A good serve of a fresh garden salad or left over salad.
One slice sourdough or pumpernickel bread depending upon which stage of the eating plan you are following. Serves 1.

Chicken and Vegetable Soup

4 chicken drumsticks, remove skin and fat
2 cups carrot, grated
½ cup parsley, chopped
1 cup parsnip, grated
1 cup swede, grated

1 cup celery, grated
One 400g can whole corn, including liquid
1 large onion, chopped & browned in a pan
Place all ingredients in a large pan and barely cover with water. Bring to boil and simmer for one hour until tender. Remove chicken bones leave meat in soup. Season with lemon pepper or cracked black pepper and sea salt to taste. Suitable to freeze in serving portions. Serves 6 to 8.

★ Grilled Fish with Peas and Pepper Salad

1 fillet of fresh fish of your choice per person - grilled
Salad – served hot or cold
1/2 cup fresh or frozen peas
1 red pepper, de-seeded and cut into strips
celery and carrot sticks
1 tbsp sesame seeds
Season of black pepper & sea salt
Simmer or steam peas and red pepper until just tender – drain and toss with sesame seed and dress with cold pressed olive or flaxseed oil and apple cider vinegar or fresh lemon juice. Serve with sticks of celery and carrot. Salad serves 2.

Prawns and Mango Salad

6 large prawns, cooked and peeled
1 cup mixed lettuce leaves
1 tomato, cut into bite size pieces
1 small Lebanese cucumber, thinly sliced
½ small red onion, sliced
1 medium mango, sliced
handful snow peas
bean sprouts to garnish
Dressing:
½ cup soy mayonnaise
1 tbsp tomato paste
1 tbsp Worcestershire sauce
½ tsp Tabasco sauce
½ tsp Horseradish sauce
1 pinch of ground oregano
Mix dressing ingredients together in a bowl with a whisk, until well combined. Store left over dressing in screw top jar or bottle in fridge. Place all salad ingredients on serving plate. Top with prepared prawns and drizzle with dressing. Serves 2 to 3.

Frittata with lettuce cups of salad

3 large eggs, lightly beaten
2 cups mixed vegetables of your choice, chopped and cooked until almost tender, ie, cauliflower, broccoli, corn, spring onions, potato, pumpkin, mushrooms, beans, peas, carrot and zucchini
2 tbsp parsley, chopped
2 tbsp soy mayonnaise
ground black pepper and sea salt to taste.
Rub a little cold pressed olive oil around a non-stick frypan.
Mix all ingredients together and pour into pan. Cook over medium heat gently until mixture is set – usually 5-7 minutes, depending on thickness of mixture. Mixture should be brown on bottom, excessive heat will burn bottom before mixture is set. Now pop pan under hot grill, just long enough to brown top. Let stand in pan for a few minutes to settle and firm up. Slice and serve warm, with lettuce cups containing any leftover salad, or a mixture of grated carrot and beetroot and sliced tomato. Serves 3.

Lentil patties with stir-fry vegetables or tossed green salad

1 cup red lentils
2 cups water
1 packet Dutch Curry Soup
A little cold pressed olive oil for cooking
1 egg lightly beaten
1 tbsp crunchy natural peanut butter
1 tbsp sesame seeds
Rinse lentils under running water, then place in pan with new water, bring to the boil and simmer for about 15 minutes or until all water is absorbed. Blend or process lentils and soup mix until smooth. Add peanut butter and sesame seeds and mix well. Refrigerate mixture for about 30 minutes to firm up. Shape into about 6 to 8 patties with floured hands. Heat oil in non-stick pan and cook patties about 4 to 5 minutes on each side or until nicely browned.
Serve patties with stir-fried vegetables, or a fresh green salad.
Freeze any leftover patties, to thaw and heat for a future meal. Serves 3.

Audrey Tea Hint

It is a good idea to check your fridge contents every couple of days so that you don't spoil or waste anything. This is a good time to do a stir-fry. Cut any vegetable of your choice into shreds or julienne stirps, put a little cold pressed olive oil in frypan and gently toss the vegetables for a couple of minutes. Pour in a little soy or oyster sauce and season to taste.

Weekend BBQ lunch with salads

Prepare ahead 3 to 4 salads from the salad selection in this book. Make enough for your family and guests. Prepare the salads that will keep in the fridge for a day or so, then you can have leftovers the next day.

For the barbecue allow per person –

1 lentil patty (today you can call it a burger)

1 piece lean minute steak, thinly sliced and sprinkled with ground oregano & lemon juice

1 chicken drumstick – skinned, or chicken kebab marinated in soy and honey.

The meat can be prepared and refrigerated a couple of hours before guests arrive.

Chicken marinade

Slightly warm and mix together 2/3 cup soy sauce, 1/3 cup honey, 1 tbsp peanut butter. Coat the chicken and leave to stand for about 1 hour. Drumsticks can be cooked in a pan in the oven until tender. Kebabs go on the BBQ with the steak and burgers. Serve meat with salads and finish off with a nice mixed fruit platter.

Tasty bean and olive salad

400g Cannelloni beans or soybeans (canned or cooked), washed and drained

3 to 4 vine-ripened tomatoes (or sun-dried tomatoes), chopped

100g black de-seeded olives, roughly chopped or halved

¼ cup pepitas (green pumpkin seeds)

¼ cup pine or pistachio nuts

Sprinkle of black cracked pepper

1 tbsp fresh basil leaves, roughly chopped

1 clove garlic, crushed

¼ cup lemon juice

1 tbsp finely grated lemon rind

A drizzle of cold pressed olive oil

Sprinkle of raw sugar or tiny pinch of stevia powder

If using fresh tomatoes, brush with cold pressed olive oil and bake uncovered in a moderate to hot oven for about 30 minutes taking care not to burn. Cool and chop roughly. Place all ingredients into a bowl and toss to gently combine. A large serve is a meal on its own. Leftovers can be stored in a sealed container in the fridge and used as a salad with meat or fish. Serves 4 to 6.

★ Coleslaw salad

This salad is simple to prepare and easy to take to work for lunch. It is nice and light served with a can of drained crabmeat or left over roast meat.

Toss all together:

¼ cabbage – Chinese or savoy are best, shredded
6 spring onions, chopped or finely sliced
1 small red chilli, de-seeded and finely chopped (optional)
½ cup fresh mint, coarsely chopped
1 cup parsley, coarsely chopped
¼ cup coriander, coarsely chopped

Dressing

¼ cup fresh lemon juice
1 tbsp Dijon mustard
½ cup cold pressed sesame or olive oil.

Mix ingredients in a screw top jar and keep in refrigerator. Dressing can be added just before serving, or in the morning if more convenient, to take to work. Serves 4 to 6.

Vegetable and Bean Soup

1 red onion, chopped
1 to 2 cloves garlic, crushed
One 400g can red kidney beans or soybeans – drained
½ cup pearl barley
400g pumpkin, peeled & chopped
4 medium zucchini, sliced
1 large carrot, sliced
One 400-425g can tomatoes
2 or more stems of celery, chopped
1 tbsp toasted sesame seeds
A drizzle of cold pressed olive oil

Heat oil in pan and brown onion and garlic until soft. Place all ingredients into large pan and barely cover with water – about 1 litre. Bring slowly to boil then simmer gently with lid on for 30 minutes, or until all vegetables are tender. If preferred you may blend or process this soup until smooth. Sprinkle with chopped parsley and toasted sesame seeds to serve. Freeze any leftovers. Serves 6 to 8.

★ Devilled eggs with olives and sprouts

2 eggs hard boiled
¼ cup soy mayonnaise
½ tsp seeded mustard
1 tsp fresh chives, chopped
few drops of Tabasco sauce
pinch of paprika & cracked black pepper & sea salt
Cut eggs in half lengthways and remove yolk. Mash egg yolks then stir in all other ingredients. Spoon the mixture back into the egg halves and serve with a mix of snow pea sprouts, onion sprouts and alfalfa sprouts and about 6 seeded black olives. Can also serve in lettuce cups, which would make an easy lunch box meal for work. Serves 1 to 2.

Easy in a rush lunch (when feeling lazy)

Two slices of sour dough, wholegrain or pumpernickel bread
Two vine-ripened tomatoes
1 tbsp cold pressed olive oil
Cracked black pepper and sea salt
Toast bread and then drizzle olive oil over the toasted bread. Layer bread with slices of freshly cut tomato. Sprinkle with pepper and salt.
Eat this with one can of sardines or crabmeat, or a drink made with unsweetened soymilk and one tbsp Synd-X protein powder. Serves 1 to 2.

★ BBQ Chicken Salad

2 cups lettuce, torn into pieces
1 tomato, sliced
½ cucumber, sliced
½ avocado, diced
½ cup mung beans, washed
chunks of barbecue chicken, remove skin and fat
½ cup kidney beans or soy beans, cooked or canned
Combine all ingredients and dress with olive oil, apple cider vinegar or lemon juice
Serves 2

★ Tuna or Salmon salad

One 210g can tuna or salmon in oil or brine
1 cup lettuce, torn
½ cup celery, chopped
½ tomato, sliced
¼ cucumber, sliced

2 spring onions, sliced
1 boiled egg, quartered
Combine all ingredients and add dressing of cold pressed olive or flaxseed oil and apple cider vinegar, or lemon juice. Serves 2.

★ Vegetarian Burger

½ cup soybeans (canned or cooked) or tofu
1 egg
½ cup peanuts
½ cup toasted sesame seeds
1 onion, finely chopped or grated
½ carrot, grated
1 stalk celery, chopped
2 cloves garlic, crushed
½ tsp dill seed, ground
salt and pepper
Preparation
Mix all ingredients with beaten egg
Add ½ tsp salt and cracked black pepper and dill seed
Shape into patties
Warm olive oil in pan and brown patties on both sides, or bake until dry and brown
Serve with fresh salad.
Serves 1 to 2

★ Vegetable and prawn stir-fry

700g uncooked king prawns
1 tbsp cold pressed olive oil
1 onion, cut into wedges
200g broccoli, cut into small pieces
2 cloves garlic, crushed (optional)
1 red capsicum, sliced
150g small mushrooms
2 tsp fresh ginger, grated
1 and ½ cups chicken or fish stock
1 and ½ tbsp lime juice
1 and ½ tbsp chilli sauce (add a pinch of stevia powder to sweeten if desired)
1 tbsp fish sauce
1 and 1/3 cups (270g) brown rice (Do not eat the rice if you are on stage one of the eating plan)

Preparation:

Peel and de-vein prawns, wash

Heat 2 tsp oil in pan or wok

Add prawns and stir-fry over high heat for 1 minute, or until browned, remove.

Heat remaining oil, add capsicum, onion and broccoli, stir-fry for 2 minutes

Add mushrooms, garlic and ginger, stir-fry for 1 minute

Add prawns and remaining ingredients, stir-fry for 2 minutes, or until tender.

Serve with boiled rice and a fresh green salad.

Serves 4

PREPARATION OF STOCKS

- The best vegetables for stock are carrots, leeks, onions (with skin), parsley stalks, celery (not the leaves), celeriac, and sweet corn.
- To add a delicious full body flavour to your stocks, try roasting the vegetables first in the oven, then place them in the saucepan and continue as per recipe
- Wash all your produce to ensure it is free from bacteria and dirt.
- With chicken stock, remove all the offal and wash thoroughly with cold running water.
- Fish stock only needs to be cooked for approximately 20 minutes, as it can become gluey.

All the stocks in this book make approximately 5 litres (20 cups) of stock

VEGETABLE STOCK

Ingredients:

2	medium onions, cut in half (do not peel)
2	large carrots, chopped in three
1/2	head celery (leaves removed)
2cm	knob of fresh ginger, sliced
6cm	stick kombu seaweed (optional)
1	bay leaf

7	black pepper corns
2tbsp	cold pressed olive oil

cups of (preferably filtered) water

Preparation:

Place oil into large saucepan on high heat, do not burn
Place all other ingredients (except water) into the pan
Stir until the smell of the vegetables releases
Add the water and bring to the boil, then simmer gently for approx. 1 hour
Strain the liquid
Toss away the solids and keep what you need
Pour into containers when cool and freeze

FISH STOCK

Ingredients:

Make sure your fish smells pleasant and don't use oily fish (such as sardines, mackerel or any smoked fish)

4	prawn heads or 1 large fish head
1	bunch coriander
1	bunch parsley
2	large onions
4	cloves garlic
6cm	stick kombu seaweed (optional)
24	cups filtered water

Preparation:

Place all ingredients in a large saucepan and bring to the boil
Skim off any scum
Return to a gentle simmer for 20 minutes
Strain and throw away all the solids
Allow to cool and remove any fat that comes to the surface
Freeze the remainder (some in small containers, as it is great to cook rice/grains etc)

CHICKEN STOCK

Ingredients:

Note: Offal can make your stock bitter

1	free-range (optional) chicken, or chicken pieces
2	medium onions, cut in quarters (skin on)
2	medium carrots, cut in half
1/2	celeriac root, peeled and halved, or 1/2 head of celery, leaves removed and halved
1	bunch parsley

1	pinch rock salt
2tbsp	cold pressed olive oil
1tsp	freshly ground black pepper (optional)
24	cups filtered water

Preparation:

Wash meat if you are using uncooked chicken
Place oil into large saucepan, on high heat, do not burn
Place all ingredients (except water and parsley) into the pan
Stir until the smell of the vegetables releases (about 5 minutes)
Add the water and the parsley
Bring to the boil (not vigorously), simmer gently for approx 2 hours
Remove solids and allow to cool
Remove fat from surface (a free-range chicken's fat is more like jelly)
Freeze remainder of stock within two days

DINNER / MAINS

The Family Roast

Roast meat can be " liver friendly" if you follow the guidelines below. Lean roasted meats are a very good source of protein for those with Syndrome X.

All of the roasts can be used as main courses for dinner and the leftovers used as cold lunchmeats. This is much healthier than using preserved delicatessen meats such as ham, devon, sausage, corn beef, smoked salmon or turkey, or fritz.

Use tender cuts of meat trimmed of all fat such as -

Scotch Fillet
Eyepiece of Silverside (not corned)
Eyepiece of Pork or Beef is an ideal cut
Leg of Lamb
Baby Veal, legs or fillet
Chicken or Turkey

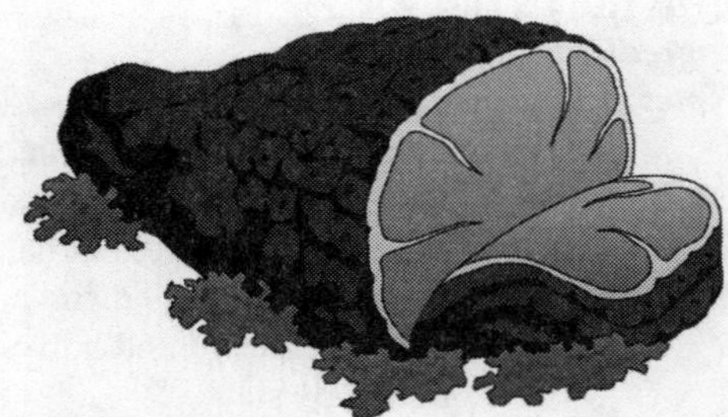

Oven Bags

Follow the directions, which come with oven bags. After the meat is prepared and placed in the oven bag, add 1 to 2 tablespoons of water to the bag, to provide the moisture to keep the meat tender and succulent. Cooking time may be slightly less than that advised on the oven bag because you will be using tender cuts of meat. Test by sliding a skewer through the bag and into the thickest part of the meat. If you prefer your roast medium rare, the juice will be pink. When the juice is clear, the roast is cooked to medium.

If you do not like using oven bags, you can achieve a similar result by roasting the meat in a covered metal baking pan, or heatproof casserole dish with a lid.

Meat will brown naturally in an oven bag. When cooking in a baking pan or casserole dish with a lid, you will have to turn and baste the meat, and leave it uncovered for the last 15mins of cooking time. If cooked without the lid for the whole of the cooking time, the meat will become very dry. This is because of the need to trim all fat prior to cooking.

Many herbs and spices can be used in preparing your roast and here are some suggestions.

★ Roast Beef

Approx. 1 and ½ to 2 kg of beef

1 dessertspoon grainy mustard

1 dessertspoon horseradish sauce

1 dessertspoon soy sauce

Mix all the ingredients to form a paste, and rub all over the meat before placing the meat in the oven bag. Cook at 200 degrees C (no higher), until the meat is cooked to your personal taste.

When the meat is cooked, remove it from the oven and snip a corner of the oven bag and retain the meat juices for gravy.

Leave the meat to stand in the oven bag before carving.

Using meat juices makes a rich gravy of your choice to pour over carved meat.

If you like garlic you can make several tiny cuts in your beef and push in slivers of fresh garlic before rubbing on spicy paste.

Serve with baked vegetables and salad.

★ Roast Lamb

Make stuffing with fresh breadcrumbs, mixed herbs and finely chopped onion or chives and just enough fruit chutney to bind mixture together. Place stuffing inside the folds of the meat and secure with skewers to hold the stuffing securely.

If on stage one of the eating plan avoid the stuffing.

Sprinkle the outside of lamb with chopped rosemary leaves, place in an oven bag with a little water and cook as directed for beef.

Serve with mint sauce and baked vegetables and salad.

★ Roast Pork

1 and ½ to 2 kg of Scotch fillet of pork

2 green apples - peeled, cored and cooked in a little water with 2 whole cloves.

When apples are cooked, remove the cloves and drain off all liquid.

To apple pulp add 1-teaspoon grainy mustard and 1/2 teaspoon dried oregano. Spread this mixture over the pork and place meat in an oven and cook as directed for beef. Apple juice can be used instead of water in the oven bag.

Serve sliced with gravy made from juices from the oven bag and your preferred gravy mixture.

★ Roast Veal

Leg of baby veal or 1 and ½ to 2-kg fillet of veal

Brush meat sparingly with soy sauce

Mix 1 packet of mushroom soup (no added sugar) with ½ teaspoon dried oregano and roll veal in this mixture until all covered.

Place meat in oven bag with 1 to 2 tablespoons of water and cook as directed for beef.

Sauce

100gm button mushrooms, sliced very thinly

2 spring onions, finely chopped

Meat juices from the oven bag made up to 1 cup with water

Cook mushrooms and onions in the liquid until just tender, then thicken with a little plain flour to make a nice pouring sauce.

Season to taste before pouring over the sliced roasted veal – delicious!

★ Roast Poultry

Buy poultry of your choice (if preferred boned and prepared), rub a few extra mixed herbs on outside of meat, and either section the bird, or place it whole, in the oven bag as directed on the oven bag. Cook until

meat is tender.
Serve with a light gravy made with meat juices (take fat off) and the flavour of your choice.
Serves 4 to 6

★ Low Fat Apricot Chicken

4 large skin-less chicken fillets - trimmed of all fat
2 tbsp chopped dried apricots
2 tbsp chopped hazelnuts
1 tsp dried oregano
Mix apricots, nuts and oregano. Cut the chicken fillets to open out as flat as possible. Lay one fillet out and sprinkle 1/3 of filling over the flesh. Repeat with each fillet until you have a stack of 4 fillets.
Sprinkle top fillet with ground black pepper and a little extra dried oregano.
Tie fillets into a parcel shape with string and place carefully into oven bag. Add 2 tablespoons of water to bag and bake in oven as directed in preparing bags for roasting.
Bake about 1 hour or until tender.
After cooking, snip bag and retain juices, make juices up to 1 cup with water, season and slightly thicken with plain flour.
Slice your chicken parcel carefully with a sharp knife and enjoy your delicious seasoned chicken topped with a tasty sauce.
Serve with steamed green vegetables and fresh salad.
Note: if you can get free range organic chicken this is more delicious
Serves 4.

★ Roast Pigeon or Quail

Buy clean and freshly dressed birds and wipe inside with paper towels
Marinade for 4 - 6 birds
1/2 cup balsamic vinegar
1/4 cup cold pressed olive oil
1/4 cup port or red wine
1 dessertspoon soy sauce
1 tsp mixed dried herbs
Mix all ingredients together and pour over birds. Cover and leave for at least an hour turning the birds occasionally.
Place birds in oven bags (you may need two bags) and pour remaining marinade in bags.
Bake at 180 degrees C for 45 minutes - test with skewer and cook for another 15 minutes if required.
Note: LSA can replace flour to thicken gravy.

Meanwhile lightly brown one chopped onion in a little oil, then add meat juices to pan and simmer until slightly thickened.
Pour over birds and serve.
Serve with roast vegetables and fresh salad.
Serves 4 - 6.

★ Rack of Lamb with lemon and rosemary

2 racks of lamb (12 chops in total)
3 cloves garlic
6 sprigs of rosemary
Juice of 1 fresh lemon
Black pepper
2 tbsp olive oil
6 sprigs Rosemary to garnish
Preparation
Preheat oven to 400 degrees C
Trim lamb of fat
Peel and halve garlic
Cut a tunnel between the meat and the bone and fill with garlic, lemon juice and some rosemary
Pierce the lamb and insert rosemary over the lambs surface.
Place racks in a baking dish, sprinkle with pepper and olive oil. Bake for 40 minutes or until cooked through. Cut rack into cutlets
Serve with steamed green vegetables and a salad.
Serves 4 to 5

★ Beef in black bean sauce

750 gr. lean rump steak – cut into strips
1 tbsp dry sherry
2 tbsp soy sauce
2 tbsp black bean sauce
1 tbsp soy flour or wholemeal flour or LSA
1/3 cup cold pressed olive oil
4 spring onions, sliced
2 stalks celery, sliced
1 red capsicum, seeded and sliced
½ cup bamboo shoots, sliced
1 tsp curry powder
Marinate beef strips in sherry, soy and black bean sauce, stir in flour and let stand for 30 minutes.
Heat oil in wok, add onions, capsicum, celery, bamboo shoots and curry

powder and sauté for 2 minutes. Remove vegetables from wok with slotted spoon.
Add meat to the remaining oil in wok and cook until browned and tender – approx 5 minutes.
Return vegetables to wok and heat through and serve with steamed carrot, broccoli and cauliflower.
Serves 4 – 6.
Green prawns can be used in place of steak for a change.

★ Quick Pork Casserole

1 medium eggplant cut into 2-cm slices
2 tbsp olive oil
900g pork fillets, cut into 2 cm cubes
1 large onion, chopped
2 cloves garlic, crushed
1 large red and green capsicum cut into 2-cm slices
810g can peeled tomatoes (no added sugar)
1 tsp dried oregano
1 tsp dried thyme
2 tsp dried basil
Preparation:
Place eggplant on a board, sprinkle with salt, and leave for 20 minutes, rinse and pat dry
Heat oil in a large pan, cook pork quickly in small batches over medium to high heat until browned. Drain on paper towels.
Add onion and garlic to pan, cook for 2 minutes
Add capsicum, cook for 4 minutes, stirring
Return pork to pan with other ingredients. Bring to boil. Simmer for about 30 minutes, stirring occasionally
Serve with a large green salad.
Serves 6

★ Spicy Pork Stir-fry

400 gr. pork fillets, trimmed of fat and cut into very thin slices
1 cucumber (leave skin on), sliced
200 gr. button mushrooms, washed
400 gr. Broccoli, chopped
1 red capsicum, finely sliced
2 tablespoon each of light soy sauce, plum sauce and hoi shin sauce
2 tbsp cold pressed olive oil
2 cups water

1/3 cup blanched almonds

Combine pork and all sauces. Refrigerate for several hours or overnight and stir occasionally.
Heat 1 tablespoon of oil in pan or wok, lift pork with a slotted spoon and add to oil. Retain marinade.
Stir and cook for about 2 minutes until meat is well browned.
Remove meat from the pan and keep warm.
Add remaining oil to pan and stir in all vegetables, cook, stirring all the time for 2 to 3 minutes. Then add the pork marinade and water and sprinkle on nuts. Return meat to the pan.
Stir over heat until mixture boils. Remove from heat and serve with chopped spring onions, steamed green vegetables, or a tossed green salad.
Serves 3 – 4

★ Marinated Indian Lamb Cutlets

16 lamb cutlets
1 tbsp grated ginger
1 tsp ground cumin
1 tsp chopped or ground coriander
½ tsp ground tumeric
½ tsp garam masala
1 tbsp lime juice
½ cup natural yogurt
3 tbsp tandoori paste
Preparation:
Trim excess fat from cutlets. Mix other ingredients in a shallow non-metallic dish.
Add cutlets and coat meat with mixture. Cover with glad wrap and refrigerate overnight. Remove cutlets from the marinade.
Brush grill with oil. Cook cutlets over medium to high heat for 4 to 5 minutes each side, or to your liking. Serve with a large green salad.
Serves 8

★ Lamb with mint and eggplant

1 medium eggplant, washed and cut into bite sized chunks
2 tbsp cold pressed olive oil
500g lean lamb fillets, thinly sliced.
2 garlic cloves, chopped
2 red chillies, de-seeded and chopped
2 tbsp fish sauce

1 tbsp tamari
1/3 cup water
30 fresh mint leaves
1 large onion, cut into thin wedges

Preparation:

Place eggplant in a colander and sprinkle with salt, leave to drain for 20minutes, rinse under cold water and drain well

Heat oil in a large pan or wok

Add lamb, onion, chillies, and garlic, cook until browned

Add eggplant and continue to cook for 5 minutes

Stir in fish sauce, tamari, water and mint leaves and heat until eggplant is softened

Serve with fresh green salad or wilted greens

Serves 4

★ Lamb and pearl barley soup

1 shoulder of lamb, trimmed of fat
3 litres of water
Salt and pepper
1 and ½ cups pearl barley
1 carrot, sliced
1 turnip, sliced
2 stalks celery, chopped
4 tbsp parsley, chopped
2 cloves garlic, finely chopped (optional)
Freshly ground black pepper.

Preparation:

Place lamb in a large pot and add water to cover. Season and bring to boil and simmer for 30 minutes, skimming the top to remove the fat.

Add barley, carrot, turnip, and celery. Simmer for 1 and ½ hours.

Remove from heat, cool and refrigerate overnight.

Remove any fat from the surface. Detach meat from the bones, cut into small pieces and return to soup.

Reheat and stir in parsley, garlic, salt and pepper and serve. Serves 6.

Creamy Chicken Curry

Chicken mixture is best-made one day ahead. Add yogurt mixture before serving.

1 kg chicken thigh fillets, fat trimmed
½ cup spelt or wheat flour

2 tsp ground cumin
¼ cup cold pressed olive oil
1 large onion, chopped
½ tsp garam masala
1 tsp curry powder (preferred strength)
½ tsp ground cumin (extra)
1 tsp ginger, grated
1 heaped tsp honey
100ml natural soy yoghurt
2 cups chicken stock
½ cup canned coconut cream
1 tablespoon lemon juice

Combine flour and cumin in a bag. Cut chicken into pieces and place in bag and shake well. Shake off excess flour.

Heat oil in large pan and brown chicken all over. Remove chicken from pan.

Add onions to pan and lightly brown and while stirring add spices, garlic, ginger and honey.

Cook for about 1 minute.

Return chicken to pan, cover, reduce heat and simmer for 45 minutes or until chicken is tender, stirring occasionally.

Yoghurt Mixture

Combine yoghurt, coconut cream and lemon juice and add to chicken, reheat but do not boil.

Serve with boiled rice and a Nice Cool Salad. Serves 6

★ Coriander and lemon chicken

2 large bunches coriander, chop leaves coarsely
2 large cloves garlic, finely chopped
5 cm piece ginger, thinly sliced
2 lemons juiced
½ tsp garam masala
1 tsp Paprika
½ tsp chilli powder (optional)
1 tsp black cumin seeds
1 tsp sea salt
1 kg chicken thigh fillets - remove fat and skin.
2 tbsp peanut oil
5 tomatoes, chopped

Preparation:

Combine coriander, garlic, ginger, lemon juice, garam masala, paprika,

chilli, cumin and salt, and mix well
Add chicken, toss well and leave in marinade for 30 minutes, stirring from time to time
Heat oil in pan, add chicken with marinade and cook over moderate heat until tender
Add tomatoes and cook for 10 minutes over low heat.
Serve with steamed vegetables and salad. Rice may be used if you have finished stage one of the eating plan.
Serves 4 to 6

★ Chicken Satay

12 chicken thigh fillets, trimmed of fat
2 tbsp chilli sauce (can use less if desired)
1 tbsp peanut oil
1 clove garlic, crushed
2 tbsp fresh coriander, chopped

Peanut sauce

250ml chicken stock
½ cup (130g) natural crunchy peanut butter
¼ cup chilli sauce (can use less if desired) – if you want sweet chilli sauce add a pinch of stevia
1 tbsp lemon juice
Combine all ingredients in a pan, simmer and stir until sauce is slightly thickened

Preparation of chicken

Cut chicken fillets into 4 strips lengthways
Combine chicken with other ingredients in a bowl and refrigerate for 3 hours, or overnight
Thread chicken strips onto skewers
Grill or BBQ until chicken is brown and tender
Serve with peanut sauce and a fresh green salad and steamed baby bok choy. Keep left-overs for lunches.

★ Goan Chicken Curry (dry)

2.5 cm fresh ginger, peeled and grated
¼ whole nutmeg, grated finely
¼ cup shredded coconut
4cloves
2.5cm cinnamon stick
1 tsp ground coriander
1 tsp ground tumeric

½ tsp cardamom seeds
½ tsp whole black peppercorns
5 cloves garlic, finely chopped
2 small red chillies, finely chopped (optional)
¾ cup water
1 large onion, finely chopped
8 skin-less chicken drumsticks
1 tsp sea salt
2 tbsp LSA

Preparation:

Toast coconut in a large, non-stick fry pan, over high heat, stirring constantly for about a minute
Add ground nutmeg, cloves, cinnamon, coriander, tumeric, cardamom and peppercorns – stirring constantly for approx 2 minutes
Place mixture into a blender, blend until finely ground
Transfer mixture into a bowl
Heat 1 tsp of the oil in a frypan
Add garlic, ginger and chillies – cook for 2 minutes
Place remaining oil in frypan, heat gently, add onion and cook until golden brown.
Stir in the chilli mixture and LSA
Add chicken, salt, spice mixture to the pan
Cook over a medium heat for 5 minutes, stirring the chicken, to cover it with the spices
Add remaining water and bring to the boil
Reduce heat, cover and simmer until the juice of the chicken runs clear – about 30 minutes
Turn the chicken frequently during cooking
Delicious served on a bed of steamed spinach (about half a bunch per person)
Serves 4

★ Fish with basil and black olives

1 tbsp olive oil
4 white fish fillets (ensure free of bones)
750g spinach, washed, trimmed and chopped
1 tbsp lemon juice
½ tsp chilli flakes or fresh chopped chilli (optional)
1/3 cup cold pressed olive oil
1 clove garlic, crushed (optional)

50g Kalamata olives
¼ cup basil leaves, shredded

Preparation:

Heat oil in large fry pan, add fish and brown on both sides until just cooked
Remove fish and keep warm
Steam spinach until just tender
Combine lemon juice, chilli, extra oil, garlic, olives and basil in same pan, cook until hot
Serve spinach topped with the fish and drizzle with oil mixture
Serve with green salad. Serves 4.

★ Poached Salmon steaks with herbs

1 cup chicken broth
½ cup water
½ tsp dill, chopped
¼ tsp dill seed
1 bay leaf
2 salmon steaks
Fresh dill and lemon slices for garnish

Preparation

Combine broth, water, bay leaf, chopped dill and dill seed in a large saucepan.
Add salmon and heat, then simmer for 4 to 5 minutes or until fish flakes easily with a fork
Place salmon on plates, garnish with fresh dill and lemon slices
Serve with mixed garden salad and dressing of cold pressed olive or flaxseed oil, and fresh lemon juice.
Serves 2

★ Stir-fry Chicken and Vegetables

2 chicken breasts (or 2 thighs per person), cut into strips
1 stalk lemon grass, remove outside layers to the soft core, and chop finely
1 tsp coarsely ground black peppercorns
2 small chillies, de-seeded and finely chopped (optional)
2 cm fresh ginger, peeled and finely chopped
2 lime leaves, finely chopped
2 limes juiced
4 tbsp tamari sauce
2 cups broccoli, chopped into bite sized pieces

1 and ½ cups green beans, washed
½ cup carrot cut into thin strips
1 onion cut into eights
1 cup small mushrooms, rinsed and halved
4 fresh coriander roots, washed and finely chopped
1 large clove garlic, finely chopped (optional)
2 tbsp cold pressed olive or flaxseed oil

Preparation:

Heat oil in wok or large fry pan
Add chicken, stir until cooked and remove from pan
Add chillies, ginger, coriander root, garlic, lemon grass, peppercorns and lime leaves to the pan and stir
Add the vegetables and lime juice and tamari, stir until almost cooked
Add chicken and stir until blended through the vegetables

★ Lemon Chicken Hotpot

1 kg skin less chicken thighs or breast fillets
2 tbsp wholemeal flour
1 tsp lemon pepper or cracked black pepper and sea salt
1 tsp curry powder

Mix flour and spices in a plastic bag, add chicken pieces and shake well.

Heat 1 tablespoon of cold pressed oil in a pan and brown chicken. Then place chicken in a casserole.

Now blend together -
1 and ½ tbsp cornflour
1 and ½ cups water
1/4 cup fresh lemon juice
1 dessertspoon sweet chilli sauce (or hot chilli sauce and a pinch of stevia powder)
1 tsp soy sauce

Stir this mixture over heat until it boils and thickens - then add 1 dessertspoon LSA and pour over chicken pieces.

Cover and cook at 200 degrees C for about one hour or until chicken is tender.

Serve with steamed broccoli and sliced carrots and a green salad.

Serves 4 - 5.

★ Cajun Fish

500g thick fish fillets – John Dory, snapper, deep sea bream, mullet, swordfish or gemfish are all suitable.

¼ cup cold pressed olive oil
2 shallots or 1 small onion, finely chopped
2 cloves garlic, minced
1 tsp sea salt
½ tsp paprika
½ tsp cayenne pepper
½ tsp freshly ground black pepper
2 tbsp chopped parsley to garnish

Cut fish fillets into 3 to 4 cm cubes.
Mix oil, onion and all seasonings together in a bowl.
Add fish pieces and stir to thoroughly coat all pieces. Let stand for at least 15 mins.
Smear some extra olive oil in a pan and heat the pan.
Add fish in a single layer and turn often until fish is cooked. Do not over cook fish. Repeat with the remaining fish. Drain fish on a paper towel.
Serve hot with a cool green salad. A squeeze of lemon juice is often a piquant addition just as you serve. My son often adds a little plain yoghurt, and lemon or lime juice to the pan juices after cooking the fish, to make a very nice spicy, creamy, piquant sauce.
Note: Cajun seasoning is available ready prepared at many supermarkets. If you prefer to use these blends, sprinkle liberally over fish before cooking in oil. Be cautious with Cajun seasonings. Hot for some can be very hot for others. Remember you can always add more seasoning if desired.
Chicken, lamb and pork are delicious prepared Cajun style.

Tuna Bake

410gm can tuna or salmon in brine, drained and broken into chunks
4 hard boiled eggs, roughly chopped
1 cup of chicken stock
½ cup soy mayonnaise
1 tsp curry powder – commercial or your own recipe
¼ teaspoon black pepper & rock salt
2 tbsp spring onions, chopped
2 cups mashed potato
1 tbsp cold pressed olive oil
Mix mayonnaise, salt & pepper, curry powder and chicken stock together in a bowl.
In a casserole dish, layer the tuna/salmon, eggs, parsley and onions.

Pour the mixture over the layers then gently spread the mashed potato over the top.
Brush the potato with a little oil, roughen the top with a fork, and bake in a moderate oven for 30 – 40 mins until heated through and the topping is a golden brown.
Serve with plenty of cooked green vegetables or a green salad of your choice. Serves 3.
Another option is to replace the tuna or salmon with an equivalent amount of canned crabmeat or shrimps.

Cooking Meat

Any meat, poultry or fish, trimmed of all fat, will give you a complete protein meal.
You can cook all of these meats by any method you choose, except for deep-frying.
If using a pan, use a non-stick variety and just oil with a little cold pressed olive oil.
All types of flavours can be added to the meats to enhance flavour. Here are some examples.

★ Lamb chops, fillets or cutlets

Sprinkle with ground oregano and a squeeze of lemon and leave to stand for ½ hour before cooking.
Spread lightly with tomato paste and sprinkle with a mixture of dried crushed basil and ground black pepper.
Drizzle with a little cold pressed olive oil and sprinkle lightly with chilli powder or sweet chilli sauce (or even better, a hot chilli sauce with a pinch of stevia powder).
Sprinkle with dried rosemary and lemon juice.

★ Beef steaks and fillets

Marinate for ½ hour in a mixture of honey, soy sauce and a dollop of natural peanut butter.
Press with cracked black pepper.
Spread with grainy mustard.
Marinate for ½ hour with a mixture of equal quantities of plum sauce, Worchester sauce, and chilli sauce.
Sprinkle with Italian or Cajun spices and a squeeze of lemon juice.
Spread with minced garlic and horseradish.

★ Pork steaks, chops, fillets and spare ribs

Spread with a mixture of grainy mustard and apple sauce.

Spread with a mixture of soy sauce, honey and cracked black pepper.
Marinate for ½ hour in plum sauce with a pinch of curry powder.

★ Chicken fillets, drumsticks and wings

Marinate in soy sauce with some honey and sesame seeds added.
Sprinkle with lemon pepper and dried parsley, which are then rubbed and pressed into the meat.
Sprinkle with mixed herbs, which are then rubbed and pressed into the meat.
There are many prepared marinades and spice mixtures that can be used, but try to choose those free of added sugar. If you prefer, just trim the meat of all fat and cook it how you choose with no additives.
Serve with some of your salad of choice and top with your favourite salad dressing.

Casserole cooking

Casserole cooking is easy and convenient.
Brown some onions in a little cold pressed olive oil. Brown the meat of your choice before putting it into a casserole dish with as many vegetables as you choose.
Add a can of tomatoes or stock, cover and cook in a moderate oven until the meat is tender.
If you roll the meat in LSA before browning, it will help thicken the juices.
You can also drain a can of soy, kidney or cannelloni beans and add them to the casserole.
Casseroles freeze very well, so always make enough for a couple of meals to save you time in the future.

RICE DISHES

Rice is easy to digest and is free of gluten. Its nutritional value is greater when unpolished (brown). There are many varieties of rice: long and short grain, sticky, glutinous, brown, white, red, black and wild.
Washing your rice until the water is clear makes it fluffy and helps to stop big clumps forming. If using the reduction method of cooking in a saucepan or a rice cooker, always separate the grains before serving with a fork. Using a spoon also stops the rice from sticking together.
A rice cooker can be a fantastic addition to any household. They can be obtained from most large department stores and Asian grocery stores. Rice cookers can be used to make delicious one pot meals (no washing up).

Try using a homemade vegetable or chicken stock to cook your rice instead of water. It's fantastic!

Spiced Rice

Ingredients:

2tbsp	cold pressed olive oil
1	onion, peeled and diced
2	cups basmati rice, cleaned washed and drained well
1	stick of cinnamon
1/2 tsp	sea salt
1tsp	cumin seeds
1	cup fresh green peas
4tbsp	sunflower seeds (dry roasted)
4 tbsp	crushed almonds
3	cups stock

Preparation:

Heat a heavy pan with a tight fitting lid and add the oil
Sauté the onions, cinnamon, almonds and cumin until golden brown
Pour in the rice and stir gently to coat the rice in the oil for about 5 minutes
Bring the stock to a simmer in a separate saucepan
Add the simmering stock to the rice and cover with the lid
Turn the heat to very low and cook for 20 minutes
Take off heat altogether
Add the peas, replace the lid immediately – leave for 5 minutes
Remove the lid and allow to stand for another 5 minutes
Fluff the rice with a metal fork (stops clumping)
Sprinkle with the dry roasted sunflower seeds
Serve as a side dish to meat, or is delicious on its own
Serves 5

Congee

Ingredients:

2	handfuls short grain rice
4	cups chicken or vegetable stock
8	thin slices of fresh ginger, 4 slices to be cut into slithers for serving with the meal
3	spring onions, finely chopped
1/4tsp	toasted sesame oil per serving

1tsp	sea salt
4	cups of chicken or fish, cut into thin strips

Preparation:

Wash the rice until the water runs clear

Mix together the stock, salt and half the ginger in a large saucepan

Add rice, mix well and bring to the boil

Reduce to a simmer as low as possible (you can use a heat diffuser)

Cook for about 30 minutes

While rice is cooking

Add ½ cm water to fry pan, bring to simmer

Add strips of chicken or fish

Cover with lid and simmer for 2 minutes, or until tender

Stir chicken/fish into rice

Serve in deep bowls topped with the remaining ginger, spring onions and toasted sesame oil

Serves 6

SOYBEAN DISHES

SOYBEANS - served in any way (as cooked beans, tempeh or tofu) with rice and seeds or nuts, make a good source of first class of protein. Tempeh and tofu both have quite a mild flavour. Tempeh will take on any flavour you cook it with, so it makes a great additive to any dish. Tempeh can be used as a meat substitute for most dishes that use meat. It can also be blended or liquidised and used in sauces, dips and dressings. When made at home, tempeh can be made from different varieties of nuts and beans.

Tempeh Curry

Ingredients:

250g	raw tempeh
2	large onions cut into wedges
1	bunch fresh coriander (wash plant, separate root from leaves, keep leaves for garnish)
600g	Jap pumpkin, cut into medium wedges, remove skin if desired
¼ cup	toasted sesame seeds
2 tsp	red or green curry paste
2 tbsp	tamarind paste (adds a tang)
400ml	coconut milk (canned)
400ml	vegetable stock

2 tbsp	cold pressed vegetable or nut oil
2	lemons - cut each lemon into 3 pieces

Cooked rice for 6 persons

Preparation:

Heat the oil in a wok or pan

Stir-fry the tempeh until golden brown and set aside

Add 1 tbsp new oil

Sauté the onions until brown

Add the washed & chopped coriander root, cook for 5 minutes

Add pumpkin and stir into the mixture

Stir the tempeh in gently

Add tamarind paste, coconut milk and stock and bring to a simmer

Cook uncovered until the pumpkin is tender and simmer to reduce the liquid

Serve on brown rice, garnish with lemon wedges and coriander leaves and sprinkle with sesame seeds

Serves 6

Chickpeas and Rice

The fresh chickpeas give this dish a delicious crunch

Ingredients:

400g	cooked chickpeas, drained and rinsed
400g	cooked rice
2-3tbsp	cold pressed olive oil
2	large garlic cloves, peeled and crushed
2tbsp	dry roasted sunflower seeds
1	red onion, finely chopped
4cm	fresh ginger, grated
1 & ½	finely grated lemon skins, then juice flesh of lemon
1	bunch coriander, washed and chopped
200g	fresh or frozen peas
1	pinch dried chilli flakes (optional)
1tsp	ground cumin
1tsp	sweet paprika

Preparation:

Heat 2 tbsp of the oil in a large frying pan

Add onion, garlic and grated ginger and cook for 5 minutes

Add chickpeas, chilli flakes and lemon rind and stir for about 30 seconds

Add lemon juice

Mix in the rice and fresh peas and stir for 1 minute and allow to cook until nearly all the juice is gone
Add coriander, cumin and paprika
Serve in a warmed bowl with a large green salad
Serves 4

Couscous and Vegetable Casserole

Ingredients:

¼ cup	cold pressed olive oil
2	brown onions, peeled and thinly sliced
4	cloves garlic, peeled and crushed
1 to 2	birds eye chillies whole (optional)
3 tbsp	tomato paste
1litre	vegetable stock or water
½	bunch coriander, washed and chopped
½	bunch parsley, washed and chopped
3	large tomatoes, quartered
2 cups	hard vegetables such as potato, carrot, fennel, swede, turnip, parsnip etc., chopped bite size pieces
2	cups of soft vegetables such as eggplant, squash, green beans, zucchini, peas etc., chopped into bite size pieces
1	lemon, the skin finely grated, then juiced
1	serve of cooked couscous per person
5tbsp	sunflower seeds and pine nuts, dry roasted
ground spices	
1tsp	cumin
1tsp	all spice
1tsp	tumeric
1tsp	sweet paprika
1tsp	black pepper
½ tsp	ginger

Preparation:

Heat oil in large pot and add onions, chilli and garlic and stir-fry for 3 minutes
Add tomato paste and spices and cook for a further 3 minutes
Add stock and water, coriander, parsley and tomatoes plus all hard vegetables
Cover & cook for about 20 minutes, then turn down heat and simmer
Add soft vegetables and cook until tender

Serve on warm couscous sprinkled with sunflower seeds and pine nuts
Serves 6-8

Fish fillets with Couscous

400g	fresh white fish fillets (ensure free of bones)
1 cup	couscous
1 cup	boiling vegetable stock
12	green beans
1	red capsicum, sliced
¼ cup	pine nuts, toasted
2 tbsp	parsley, chopped
6	black olives halved

Preparation

Warm olive oil in pan and add fish and cook
Place couscous into a bowl and pour over boiling stock
Cover and leave for 5 minutes
Cook beans and capsicums until just tender
Fluff up couscous with a fork
Add pine nuts, parsley, olives and vegetables
Serve fish on top of couscous
Serves 2

★ Spiced Prawns

500g	uncooked medium-king prawns
1 tsp	tumeric
1 tsp	ground cumin
2	cloves garlic, crushed
1 tbsp	lemon juice
1 tbsp	cold pressed olive oil

Preparation:

Shell and devein prawns, rinse prawn meat
Combine all other ingredients, add prawns, and stir
Refrigerate for one hour
BBQ or grill prawns for 2 minutes each side
Serve with steamed green vegetables and fresh salad
Serves 2

★ Lemongrass and Tofu

This is great for BBQ's or on the grill
Ingredients:

375g	firm tofu, cut into 24 cubes

2	cloves garlic, peeled & crushed
1	knob fresh ginger, grated
2tbsp	soy sauce or tamari
2tbsp	cold pressed olive or sesame oil
1	stick of lemongrass, cut off roots (peel the first 2 layers off) and chop finely
½ tbsp	sesame seeds
1	red capsicum, de-seeded & cut into 8 cubes
2	medium zucchini, wash and trim ends
2	medium Japanese eggplants, wash and trim ends
8	dry lemongrass stalks (to be used as skewers) or use regular skewers
½ cup	sesame seeds, toasted
½ cup	pine nuts or peanuts, toasted or raw
	freshly ground black pepper

Preparation:

Toss tofu, garlic, ginger, soy sauce, oil and chopped lemongrass

Set aside to marinate

Slice the zucchini into 2, then cut each piece into 4

Repeat for the eggplant, make the slices smaller so you have 24 pieces altogether

Sprinkle the eggplant pieces with salt and leave to stand for 30 minutes

Drain the juices from the eggplant and pat dry with paper towel

Cut roots off lemongrass, peel off the hard outer leaves

Skewer one piece of capsicum, zucchini and tofu, three of eggplant, one of tofu, zucchini and one more tofu

Repeat with the remaining skewers (if the lemongrass is too flexible to pierce the firm vegetables, use a regular skewer)

Drizzle remaining marinade over the top and season with salt and pepper

BBQ or char grill until golden brown for about 20 minutes

Serve with toasted sesame seeds and nuts and a green leafy salad

Makes 8 large skewers

Tempeh with Chinese Greens and Noodles

Ingredients:

5tbsp	cold pressed sunflower oil
2	medium onions, cut into 8 pieces
3	cloves garlic (optional)
1tbsp	freshly grated ginger
1	birdseye chilli, finely chopped (optional)
2tbsp	salted black beans, soaked in boiling water for 1/2 hour (optional)
6	shiitake mushrooms, soaked in boiling water for 10 mins or until soft, keep mushroom liquid, and finely slice mushrooms
500ml	stock (vegetable or chicken)
3tbsp	mirin (is a golden liquid made from brown rice) - optional
6tbsp	soy sauce or tamari
2tbsp	kudzu or cornflour dissolved in cold water
1	bunch bok choy
1	bunch choy sum (can be replaced with other green vegetables)
1	bunch gaii choy (Chinese mustard greens)
1	bunch Chinese broccoli
1	head broccoli, wash, cut into small florets, including stalk
500g	fresh rice noodles, thick or thin
375g	tempeh, cut in half, then into thin slices
3tbsp	sunflower seeds, dry roasted
3tbsp	pine nuts or peanuts, toasted

If more convenient all the Asian greens in this recipe could be replaced with other green vegetables – green beans, broccoli, snow peas, spinach etc.

Preparation:

Heat saucepan and add 3 tbsp oil and warm
Add tempeh, cook for 2 minutes
Sauté onion until soft and lightly brown
Add garlic, ginger and chilli, cook for three minutes
Add drained beans and sliced mushrooms and stir
Stir in 450ml of stock, with mirin, mushroom water and half the soy sauce/tamari
Simmer for 10 minutes
Stir in kudzu or cornflour to thicken, cook another three minutes
Remove from heat and set aside

Preparation of noodles

Trim greens and wash very well
Heat large fry pan, add 1 tbsp oil
Toss in broccoli, till bright green
Add greens, stems first, till wilted
Toss in leaf ends, cook another 3 minutes
Place on serving plate
reheat pan and add remaining oil and then rice noodles
Cook on high heat until they soften and begin to brown and crisp on the bottom
Add remaining soy, stock and cook for a further 3 minutes
Remove from the heat, place on plate
Pour hot black bean sauce over the greens and noodles
Sprinkle seeds and nuts over the top
Serves 6

Grilled Swordfish with Olive Tapenade and Garlic Mash

Ingredients:

6	fillets swordfish (can substitute flathead, blue eye cod or Atlantic salmon)
120g	black or green olive tapenade see recipe page__
8	large potatoes, peeled
2	garlic cloves, peeled and finely chopped
1-2tbsp	cold pressed olive oil
1	splash of soy/rice/milk

Freshly ground pepper and sea salt
Enough plain flour for coating the fish

Preparation:

Sprinkle flour onto a plate, coat one piece of fish, turn so both sides are covered and repeat for all pieces of fish
Chop potatoes into small chunks and place into saucepan of water, with chopped garlic and cookpotatoes until soft
Heat a large frypan and add some oil and the fish
Cook fish until golden brown
Drain water from the potatoes and garlic
Mash potatoes and garlic and remaining oil
Whip potatoes and garlic with a fork to fluff up
Place potato mash on serving plate in the centre
Add fish to the top of the potato
Scrape a thin layer of tapenade onto the fish
Serve with a green salad and freshly steamed asparagus
Serves 6

Miso with Silken Tofu

Note: silken tofu is very delicate, handle with care

Ingredients:

1/4	cup dried arame
5	cups water
½ packet	buckwheat noodles (cooked as per instructions on the packet)
1/2	leek, washed and cut into julienne strips
3tsp	miso
1tsp	finely grated ginger
400g	silken tofu
1	cup fresh green beans, washed and thinly sliced
Gomasio	to serve, sprinkle on to taste *(see recipe page 251)*

Preparation:

Add the arame to cook with the noodles, then drain and set aside
Bring water to boil and add leek and beans and simmer 1 minute
Remove from heat, add drained arame, noodles, miso and ginger
Stir broth constantly to dissolve miso (do not boil miso)
Cut tofu into slices and divide between four warmed bowls
Pour noodles and vegetables with the broth over the tofu
Sprinkle with Gomasio or sesame seeds and finely chopped spring onions
Serve with a fresh salad of choice
Serves 4

★ Tofu and Lotus Root Stir-fry

Ingredients:

8	dried shiitake mushrooms, soaked in warm water for 30 minutes
2tbsp	cold pressed olive oil
400g	firm tofu, cut into bite sized pieces
1	medium onion, finely sliced
8x5mm	slices frozen/fresh lotus root
1	small head of broccoli, washed and cut into florets
100g	snow peas, washed and trimmed
2tbsp	toasted sesame seeds and pine nuts or peanuts

Soy sauce to taste

Preparation:

Remove mushrooms from water, take off stems
Heat oil in a wok or frypan, add tofu and brown on both sides
Remove tofu from pan and set aside
Stir-fry onion, lotus root, broccoli, snow peas and mushrooms
Fold through tofu when vegetables are tender but still crisp
Serve with sesame seeds and toasted pine nuts and soy sauce. Side salad of fresh greens.
Serves 3 to 4

★ Lentil Fritters

Ingredients:

2tbsp	cold pressed sesame/canola oil
1	onion, finely chopped
1tsp	ground coriander
1tsp	salt
1 cup	red lentils washed and soaked in cold water for 15 mins
140ml	cold water
4tbsp	spring onions chopped roughly
5tbsp	rice powder/all purpose flour
1tbsp	cornflour/cornstarch
1	egg, beaten
1pinch	ground black pepper/white pepper

Canola oil for stir-frying

Preparation:

Heat sesame oil in a wok/frying pan
Stir-fry onions for 2 mins, add coriander, salt and lentils, and cook for another 2 mins
Add water, simmer, stirring often for approx 5 minutes until the water is absorbed
Leave to cool
Add rest of the ingredients to cooled lentils, mix well
Heat oil for stir-frying in either a wok or small saucepan
Drop heaped tablespoon of lentil mix into oil – approx 1 minute each side
Repeat until all mixture is gone
Remove from oil with a slotted spoon, drain on absorbent paper

Serve hot or cold with a big green salad and Gomasio, or steamed vegetable salad with tahini dressing
These fritters are great in lunch boxes
Makes approx 30 fritters

Calamari and Rice

Ingredients:

550g	squid cleaned and sliced into rings
Rice	
1½ cups	white long grain rice (basmati, jasmine)
2tbsp	cold pressed olive oil
2	shallots, finely chopped
2	cloves garlic, crushed
1	cinnamon stick
3	cardamom pods, preferably green
5tsp	salt
2 & 1/4 cups	fish or vegetable stock, or water
Marinade	
2tbsp	lime juice
1tsp	lemongrass, finely chopped
1tsp	chillies, (red or green) finely chopped (optional)
1tsp	parsley, finely chopped
2	cloves garlic, crushed
2tbsp	tamari or fish sauce
1tbsp	cold pressed olive oil
1	bunch coriander, washed and finely chopped

Preparation:

Mix all marinade ingredients in a bowl
Place squid in marinade and leave for 15 minutes
Heat olive oil in a saucepan and stir-fry all the rice ingredients (except the rice)
Cook for a further 3 minutes
Add stock/water, bring to the boil
Stir in the rice when the stock is boiling
Turn down the heat, stir and bring to a simmer
Simmer rice for 15 minutes, or until liquid has disappeared
Cover saucepan with lid, leave on lowest heat for 10 minutes
Drain squid and place on top of rice and cover
Increase the heat a little and leave to cook for 1 to 2 minutes
Remove pan from heat, leave covered, place on a wet folded tea towel and leave for 2 minutes

Take off lid, stir the squid through, pick out cinnamon stick and cardamom pods
Add coriander and stir through
Serve hot with wilted greens (see below) or a fresh garden salad
Serves 4-6

★ Wilted Greens

Ingredients:

1 bunch	English spinach, washed, larger stems removed
2 bunch	baby bok choy, washed, quartered length ways
1 bunch	Asian broccoli. washed, cut into finger size lengths
1tsp	lemon skin (finely grated) = lemon zest
3tbsp	tamari
1tbsp	toasted sesame seed oil or cold pressed olive oil

Preparation:

Place all greens into a saucepan with lemon zest
Heat saucepan until steaming. The water from the washed greens will be enough to steam/stir-fry greens
Warm sesame oil and tamari
Remove vegetables from the heat when they are wilted, bright green and slightly crisp
Place greens on a serving dish
Pour warmed tamari and oil over greens
Serves 2 – 6 (6 if served with another dish)

Hot Fish Curry

Ingredients:

550g	cod steaks or monk fish fillets (or ask the fish man what fish is good for curry) cut into chunks
80ml	cold pressed olive oil
3 cups	canned coconut milk
2 cups	fish stock or water
450g	small new potatoes, scrubbed and washed
Enough	cooked rice for each bowl

Curry paste

1	onion chopped
3	cloves garlic, chopped (optional)
5 cm	piece of lemongrass, chopped, outer leaves discarded
2.5cm	piece of galingale, peeled and chopped
2	Kaffir lime leaves, shredded

1tsp	ground black pepper
4-5	red chillies, de-seeded and chopped (optional)
1tbsp	roasted coriander seeds
1tbsp	roasted cumin seeds
½tsp	ground nutmeg
½tsp	ground tumeric
1tbsp	fish sauce
2tbsp	lemon juice
1tsp	salt

Note: You may use prepared curry paste

Preparation:

Heat oil in a large saucepan
Brown fish slightly in oil and set aside
Place all ingredients for the curry paste with 4 tbsp of coconut milk into a blender, blend until smooth
Pour the paste into the saucepan and bring to the boil, then simmer for 5 minutes
Add rest of coconut milk and stock or water, bring almost to the boil
Add potatoes and simmer uncovered for 20 minutes
Place fish on top of curry and continue to simmer for another 10 mins
Serve curry on top of warm or hot rice
Do not thicken the sauce as the consistency should be like a soup
Serves 4 - 6

★ Tempeh Burgers

Ingredients:

4tbsp	cold pressed olive oil
2	onions, finely chopped
3	cloves garlic, finely diced
1-2	red chillies, de-seeded and finely chopped (optional)
1tsp	ground cumin
1tsp	ground coriander
4 cups	tempeh, chopped finely or blended
2tbsp	parsley, chopped finely
2	eggs

Salt and pepper to taste

Preparation:

Heat 2tbsp oil in a fry pan
Stir-fry onions until slightly golden, add garlic, chilli, spices, cook for another minute

Stir in tempeh and pepper and salt to taste
Cook for another 2 minutes
Remove all the cooked ingredients to a bowl and leave to cool
Mix in parsley and the eggs, mix well
Form into 4-6 patties
Shallow-fry in the remaining oil in a non-stick pan, 4-6 minutes each side
Serve as a traditional burger with salad and vegetables
Serves 4-6

★ Stir-fry Tempeh with vegetables

Ingredients:

1tbsp	toasted sesame seed oil
1 tbsp	sunflower seeds
1 tbsp	sesame seeds
3tbsp	cold pressed canola or olive oil
3cm	knob of fresh ginger, grated
1	large onion, halved and roughly sliced
1	red chilli, de-seeded and thinly sliced (optional)
1/2	head broccoli, washed and cut into florets
1 cup	fresh or frozen peas
6 pieces	lotus root, halved
1 pkt	baby corn
2	handfuls of fresh green beans, washed, topped and tailed
4tbsp	tamari or light soy
2 cups	vegetable/chicken stock or water
375g	tempeh, halved length ways then thinly sliced
1 bunch	fresh coriander
1 cup	pumpkin, thinly sliced

Rice for four people
(Avoid the rice if you are on stage one of the eating plan)

Preparation:

Heat olive oil in a wok or large fry pan
Toss in ginger, chilli and onion, stir-fry for 3 minutes
Add tempeh and cook until golden brown, stirring fairly constantly
Add a splash of stock if you need to
Toss in half of coriander and all the vegetables
Pour in stock and tamari
Continue to cook on a high heat until vegetables are cooked, with a little bit of crunch

Pour toasted sesame seed oil over vegetables and stir through
Turn off heat
Serve in big deep bowls on top of rice – don't forget the delicious cooking juices for the rice
Garnish with remaining coriander, sunflower and sesame seeds
Serves 4

Vegetable Noodle Soup

Ingredients:

1 and ½	bunches of English spinach, wash & remove large stalks, tear into pieces
1/2 bunch	fresh coriander, wash & chop, including the roots
1 bunch	parsley, wash and chop, remove stems
1/2 bunch	spring onions, washed and finely chopped
100g	fettuccine, broken into pieces
750g	can of red kidney beans, or soybeans drained
1 cup	green lentils cooked until tender (or you can use a can of lentils)
1 and ½ litres	vegetable or chicken stock
2	brown onions, peel and finely chopped
3tbsp	cold pressed olive oil
1 cup	cooked rice
2 handfuls	pine nuts, toasted

Preparation:

Stir-fry brown onions until crisp in one tbsp cold pressed oil – set aside
Mix spinach, coriander, parsley and spring onions together, set aside
Heat 2tbsp cold pressed oil in a large saucepan
Place fettuccine, kidney beans, 1cup of stock, cooked lentils and garlic into the large saucepan, cook for 5 minutes
Pour in enough stock to cover the ingredients in the pan, cover and bring to the boil
Reduce heat and simmer for 15 minutes or until cooked
Add greens and stir, allowing them to wilt, then add rice and cooked onions
Simmer gently for 5 minutes
Serve in large bowls, garnished with crisp onions and pine nuts
Serves 6-8

★ Moroccan Fish

Ingredients:

2tbsp	cold pressed olive oil
1	onion, chopped
3	cloves garlic, crushed
½	medium fennel bulb, washed and thinly sliced
¼ tsp	fennel seeds
1tsp	ground cumin
500g	ripe tomatoes, washed and chopped
2tsp	sun dried tomato paste
4	blue eye cod steaks or haddock/swordfish fillets
1 bunch	parsley, washed & chopped
1	lemon, rind grated then juiced

Salt and pepper to taste

Preparation:

Heat 1tbsp oil in frying pan

Add onion, garlic, cumin, fennel and fennel seeds, stir-fry 2 to 3 minutes

Stir in tomatoes, and cook for 2 minutes

Add tomato paste, simmer for 15 minutes, stir occasionally, and set aside

Heat remaining oil in fry pan

Add fish and sear - brown quickly on both sides

Transfer fish to kitchen paper and wipe out pan to remove excess oil

Turn off the heat

Lay most of the parsley on the bottom of the pan

Place the fish in a single layer on top of the parsley

Sprinkle lemon rind and juice and season with pepper and salt

Pour over the tomato sauce, apply heat to simmer for 10 minutes

Serve with steamed green vegetables (asparagus, spinach, beans etc) and garnish with parsley. Serve a green salad on the side.

Serves 4

★ Squid with Vegetables and Herbs

Ingredients

2tbsp	cold pressed olive oil
2	onions chopped
3	cloves garlic, crushed
1	fresh red chilli, de-seeded and thinly sliced (optional)
2	anchovy fillets
300g	eggplant (aubergine), cut into 2.5cm cubes
4	mint leaves, torn
5tbsp	parsley, chopped (2tbsp for garnish)
2	smallish zucchini, sliced
4	ripe tomatoes, quartered
100g	roast capsicum, roughly chopped
1kg	squid, prepared and cut into small squares

Enough cooked rice for each plate

(Avoid the rice if you are on stage one of the eating plan)

Salt and pepper to taste

Preparation

Heat 1tbsp of the oil in a large fry pan

Add onion, garlic, chilli and cook until softened

Stir in anchovies, mash them so they can dissolve

Add eggplant and cook for 5 minutes

Toss in the mint, parsley and zucchini, allow zucchini to wilt, then

Add tomatoes and capsicum, stir occasionally, until vegetables are tender Just before serving

Heat remaining oil in another pan

Toss in the squid, stir-fry on high heat, for about 90 sec

Remove squid with slotted spoon

Place cooked rice on plates, add the vegetables, then the squid

Garnish with thinly sliced preserved lemon, or parsley

Serves 6

Rice and Mung Dal with cauliflower and peas

Ingredients:

1 cup	basmati rice
1 small	cauliflower, washed, dried and cut into small florets
2tbsp	cold pressed olive oil
1/2tbsp	fresh grated ginger
1	hot green chilli, de-seeded, finely chopped (optional)

1tbsp	cumin seeds
145g	split moong dal, without skins (or red lentils, rinsed)
180g	fresh peas (or you can use frozen peas - defrosted)
7 cups	water or vegetable stock
1½ tsp	tumeric
2 handfuls	almond flakes
1 pinch	salt

Preparation:

Wash rice until the water runs clear, generally about six rinses

Heat oil in a large saucepan, add ginger, chilli and cumin seeds, stir fry until the cumin seeds turn brown, stir constantly

Toss in the cauliflower, quickly, stir through and cook for a further 5 minutes

Stir in the rice and dal (or lentils) and cook for another minute

Pour in the fresh peas, stock and tumeric, bring to the boil

Reduce heat to low, partially cover and cook slowly for 1 and ½ hours, stir occasionally – cook until rice and dal are soft (cooking time will be less for lentils) – similar to porridge in consistency. If you are using frozen peas, add during the last 5 minutes of cooking time.

Stir frequently to stop sticking, before serving add salt

Serve in bowls garnished with flaked almond

Serve with a large green salad drizzled with a tart dressing (such as oil and fresh lemon juice)

Serves 4 to 6

Rice and Bean Hot Pot

Ingredients:

500g	red or white kidney beans or soybeans, soaked over night
2	celery stalks, washed and halved
3	bay leaves, fresh if possible
4	sprigs parsley
2tbsp	olive oil
500g	brown onions, chopped
5	cloves garlic, crushed
2	fresh chillies, fresh (optional)
2	tomatoes, chopped red capsicums, cored, de-seeded and very finely chopped

1tbsp	sweet paprika
1 bunch	altogether of mint, parsley and coriander, chopped finely
1 handful	fresh walnuts dry roasted, crushed
½ handful	fresh pine nuts dry roasted
½ handful	toasted sesame seeds
Extra	mint leaves for garnish
Cooked	rice for each plate
Kitchen string	

Sauce

2, 400gm cans	chopped tomatoes
2tsp	cold pressed olive oil
½ bunch	parsley, finely chopped

Preparation:

Beans

Boil the beans in water for 10 minutes, drain and discard the water

Tie parsley, celery and bay leaves together

Cover the beans with fresh cold water, add the herbs and simmer for 1 hour until the beans are just tender

Drain beans and keep the cooking liquid and discard the herbs

Sauce

Empty tomatoes and their juice into a saucepan

Add oil and parsley, simmer uncovered for 20 minutes, until thicker

To prepare casserole, heat oil in heavy casserole dish

Add onions, garlic, chilli, peppers, tomatoes and paprika, cook gently for approx 5 minutes

Stir in the beans, the sauce and enough of the cooking liquid to cover the beans

Season with salt and pepper, cover and cook in a pre heated oven (150C or 300F) for 30minutes, stir occasionally

Add the mint, parsley and coriander, stir through

Place warm rice in bottom of serving bowls

Serve beans on top of the rice

Garnish with dry roasted nuts and sesame seeds and a few mint leaves

Serves 8

You may freeze remainder in individual containers for another day

★ Garlic Baked Cod with Green Beans and Tomatoes

Ingredients:

4	good size pieces of blue eyed cod fillets
250gm	green beans washed, topped & tailed
1	onion, thinly sliced
6	large cloves of garlic, thinly sliced (can use less if desired)
4tbsp	parsley, washed and chopped
2tbsp	olive oil
400g	can chopped tomatoes, with juice
1tsp	fresh or dried oregano
15	black olives

Plenty of freshly ground black pepper

A little water

Preparation

Mix beans, onion, garlic, pepper and olive oil together in a roasting pan

Lay pieces of cod on top of the above mixture

Spread tomatoes over the top of the fish

Sprinkle with oregano and a bit more black pepper

Place in a pre heated oven (375F/190C) for 45 mins or until cooked

Remove 2 to 3 times to use juice to baste the fish

Add cold water if it begins to dry out too much

Toss in the black olives for the last 20 minutes of cooking time

Serves 4

Vietnamese Noodle Soup with Seafood

Ingredients:

1	small squid, cleaned and cut into bite size pieces
300g	firm fish fillet
200g	green prawns, shelled and de-veined
100g	scallops
2tbsp	canola oil
6	small stems of young Chinese broccoli, cut into 5cm lengths, peel away any tough skin
2 litres	chicken stock
300g	fresh egg noodles
3	spring onions, finely chopped
2	lemons, cut into quarters

6tsp	soy sauce or tamari (maybe more depending on taste)

Fresh chilli sliced (optional)

Preparation:

Heat stock in a large saucepan and leave on stove to simmer
Bring another large saucepan of water to the boil and add egg noodles
Cook for 2 minutes until tender, drain, keep cooking liquid
Divide noodles between 6 serving bowls
Return the noodle water to the boil, add broccoli and cook for 2 minutes
Remove broccoli with a slotted spoon, discard water
Use a small strainer to put the seafood in and dip it into the simmering chicken stock, a bit at a time, hold in the stock until cooked, about 30 sec
Distribute cooked seafood evenly among the bowls
Bring chicken stock back to the boil
Sprinkle spring onions evenly between the bowls
Pour in hot chicken stock
Serve chilli, lemons and tamari as side dishes to be added as desired. Serve with large garden salad.
Serves 6

Sweets and Treats

Soy custard

2 cups	unsweetened soy milk
1 tsp	cold pressed olive oil
2	eggs
¼ tsp	white stevia powder
½ tsp	vanilla

Warm soymilk (a heavy soymilk like Vitasoy is best) and beat in the oil
Beat eggs until frothy then add the stevia powder
While beating, add warm milk in a thin stream. Add vanilla
Pour the mixture into a greased baking dish
Place in shallow pan of water
Bake at 160°C/300° F for 40 minutes until custard is set
This custard is nice with baked or stewed fruits
Serves 2 - 4

Banana Pops

Cool and delicious on a hot day
Large strawberries can be prepared the same way.

2	passionfruit – scrape out the pulp

1 cup	natural soy yoghurt
4	bananas, ripe but firm

Chopped nuts or LSA to sprinkle
Peel bananas, cut in half crossways
Push a pop stick or bamboo skewer through centre of banana
Place in freezer until frozen hard
Mix passionfruit pulp with natural soy yoghurt and dip frozen bananas into mixture until covered, allow to drip drain
Sprinkle with chopped nuts or LSA and return to freezer
Makes 8 pops

Rockmelon pops

½	rockmelon
1 cup	natural soy yoghurt
1/2 cup	pineapple in natural juice, drained or fresh, diced (juice not required)
1 tsp	mint, fresh, finely chopped

Chopped nuts or LSA for sprinkles
Peel and de-seed half a rockmelon
Cut rockmelon into wedges of similar size to half a banana
Place a pop stick or bamboo skewer into melon wedges and freeze
Mix all remaining ingredients together
Dip frozen rockmelon into mixture until covered, allow to drip drain
Sprinkle with chopped nuts or LSA
Return to the freezer

Berry surprise

1 cup	fresh raspberries, blackberries and/or loganberries
1/8 to ¼ tsp	white stevia powder
1	orange – grate rind and then juice orange
2 tsp	gelatine, dissolved in a little hot water (or agar agar)
1 cup	natural soy yoghurt

Warm berries, stevia powder, rind and juice in a small saucepan over low heat
Add gelatine mixture and stir. Allow to cool.
Gently fold yoghurt through berry mixture
Place in 4 individual serving dishes.
Chill in refrigerator
Serve garnished with a few extra berries, sliced kiwi fruit and a small scoop of soy ice cream
Serves 4

Confetti rice

1 cup	oat, soy or rice milk
1 tbsp	honey, or 1/8th to ¼ tsp white stevia powder to sweeten as desired
½ cup	dried apricots, chopped
½ cup	natural sultanas
2 slices	dried mango, chopped
1 and ½ cups	rice cooked until tender
2 tbsp	shredded coconut

Place fluffy rice into a saucepan with all other ingredients
Mix all together over a low heat until well combined
If necessary, add more milk to gain your preferred consistency
Serve warm or cold.
If left to stand, add more milk as dried fruit will take up the moisture
Serves 4

Next best cream

A non-dairy gluten free cream, great on fresh fruit or fruit cooked in natural juices only

200 to 250gms	silken tofu
1 cup	soy milk
1 dstsp	honey or 1/8th tsp white stevia powder
1/2 tsp	pure vanilla essence
3 tbsp	arrowroot

Blend arrowroot with a little milk in a saucepan
Add remaining milk
Stir continually over medium heat until mixture thickens
Allow to cool, Add all other ingredients to thickened mixture
Beat with an electric mixer on low speed until mixture is thick and resembles whipped cream. Serve with fresh fruit or anywhere that you would use cream.
Serves 4

Quick mix coconut cake

2 cup	SR wholemeal flour
½ cup	raw sugar and ½ tsp white stevia powder
1 cup	coconut milk, tinned
3/4 cup	cold pressed olive oil
3	eggs
½ cup	shredded coconut
1	large lemon – grate the rind and juice

Mix all ingredients in a large bowl, beat for 2 to 3 minutes, until the consistency of batter
Pour mixture into a 23cm (9-inch) cake tin lined with greaseproof paper
Bake at 180°C/350°F for about 40 to 45 minutes - test with a skewer
When cool sprinkle with coconut

Audrey Tea Hint

When the cake is cold cut it into 3 bars, wrap 1 or 2 bars and freeze for later. When defrosting frozen cake, slice while still firm, as it thaws more quickly.

Oatmeal Pie Crust

2 cups	rolled oats
1 cup	hot water
½ cup	rice flour
1 tbsp	cold pressed olive oil
1 tbsp	lemon juice

Mix oats and water and bring to the boil in a saucepan, stirring constantly until mixture thickens
Stand until cold
Fold in the other ingredients and press mixture into a pie dish or 2 small pie dishes
Fill with your favourite filling
For sweet pie add 1 tbsp honey or ¼ to ½ tsp white stevia powder
For savoury pie add salt or herbs to taste

American Pumpkin Pie

cups	pumpkin (butternut/blue) – cook, mash and drain
1 cup	soft tofu
1 and ½ tsp	cinnamon
½ tsp	ground ginger or freshly grated
½ tsp	ground nutmeg
¼ cup	soy, rice or oat milk
½ cup	honey or ½ tsp white stevia powder
1 tbsp	orange rind grated
½ cup	pecans or walnuts, chopped

Blend all ingredients except nuts, in a food processor until smooth
Pour mixture into 23cm (9-inch) pie dish, lined with uncooked pie crust
Sprinkle top with nuts
Bake in a moderate oven for 35 to 40 minutes until golden and set
Garnish with any fresh fruit – kiwi fruit looks nice
Serve with next best cream if desired
Serves 4

Carrot and apple cake

1 cup	wholemeal SR flour
¼ cup	honey or maple syrup, and ¼ to ½ tsp white stevia powder
3/4 cup	pecans or walnuts chopped
1 cup	carrot, grated
1 cup	granny smith apple grated, leave on skin
2 tbsp	cocoa
1/2 tsp	bicarb soda
2	eggs

Sift flour, cocoa and soda into large bowl
Mix in beaten eggs and all other ingredients and combine well
Spoon mixture into a greased ring tin
Bake in a moderate oven for 40 - 45 minutes or until cooked
Test with a skewer, cool in tin
Serve dusted with a little cinnamon

Syndrome X Energy Cookie

½ cup	cold pressed olive or flaxseed oil
3 tbsp	golden syrup
1	egg beaten
1tsp	vanilla essence
1 and ½ cups	plain wholemeal flour sifted with 1 tsp bicarb soda
1 cup	sultanas and raisins or mixed fruit
1 cup	raw muesli – *see recipe page 255*
½ cup	roasted peanuts
½ cup	pepitas
1 tbsp	LSA

Mix all dry ingredients together in a large bowl.
Warm oil and syrup together to blend and then add to dry ingredients with the beaten egg.
Place large teaspoons of mixture on a tray lined with baking paper and slightly flatten.
Cook in oven at 160 degrees C for 12 to 15 minutes or until light brown. Cool on tray then on wire rack until cold.
Store in airtight container.
Makes about 60 cookies.
Have 2 to 3 cookies per snack.

Syndrome X Energy Slice

This slice is unbelievably tasty, nutritious and energy boosting

1 cup	natural sultanas
1 cup	dates chopped
1 cup	dried apricots chopped
1 cup	mixed nuts chopped – almond, cashews, brazils or pecans
½ cup	sunflower seeds
½ cup	pepitas
3cups	freshly squeezed orange juice
1 tsp	mixed spice

Put all ingredients in a saucepan and heat slowly until just simmering. Remove from heat to cool.

When cool put into a large bowl with –

¾ cup	LSA
1 and ½ cups	wholemeal SR flour
2	large beaten eggs

Spread evenly into lamington tin lined with baking paper

Sprinkle top with ¼ cup sesame seeds

Press seed down firmly and bake in medium oven at 150 degrees C for 45 minutes to one hour, or until cooked when tested with skewer

Cool in tin.

Using a sharp knife cut into fingers and store in airtight container

Note: Brazil nuts are ideal for this recipe and provide extra selenium.

Light and lovely bananas

4 large	bananas, peeled, sliced lengthways then crosswise
1 cup	orange juice, freshly squeezed
1/2 cup	lemon juice, freshly squeezed
1 tbsp	orange rind or zest
2 tbsp	honey or 1/8th tsp white stevia powder
1 tsp	cinnamon
3	passion fruit (pulp only)

Place juices, stevia (or honey) and rind in a large flat pan and heat until it simmers

Add cinnamon, then add sliced bananas and cook for 1 to 2 minutes

Remove immediately to serving comport

Spoon over juices and top with passionfruit

Serves 4

Tangy and spicy apple bake

2	large green apples, peeled and cored
3 tbsp	lemon or orange juice
1 tsp	lemon or orange rind, grated
2 tbsp	honey or ¼ tsp white stevia powder
1 tbsp	raisins or natural sultanas
8	dried apricots
8	prunes, pitted
1/2 tsp	cinnamon, ground

Slice apples into thin wedges
Toss in juice and arrange wedges around the edge of a casserole dish
Combine the juices with the rind, honey and dried fruits
Sprinkle through the cinnamon
Place this mixture through the centre of the casserole
Cover with foil
Bake in a moderate oven for 30 minutes or until apple is tender
Serve warm, topped with soy yoghurt
This dish can be prepared a few hours ahead and warmed before serving
Serves 4

Baked winter fruit salad

2 large	green apples, peeled and thinly sliced
2 large	pears, peeled and thinly sliced
1 tsp	cinnamon, ground
2 tbsp	honey or 1/8th tsp white stevia powder
1/2 cup	raisins, seeded
1/2 cup	almonds, blanched and sliced
1 tbsp	orange peel , shredded
1 small	tin unsweetened crushed pineapple, drained, keep juice

Mix together pineapple, honey (or stevia), raisins, cinnamon and peel
Place 1/3 of apples and pears overlapping, in a deep 23cm (9-inch) pie dish
Top with 1/2 of the mixture
Place another 1/3 layer of apple and pear slices
Top with remaining half of mixture
Finish with the apple and pear layer
Pour remaining pineapple juice over the fruit.
Cover dish and bake in a moderate oven for 45 minutes

Remove cover, shake a little extra cinnamon over top and sprinkle the almond slices
Serve warm with a dollup of next best cream
Serves 6.

Pear truffles

Serve these with coffee after a leisurely dinner

1 cup	pears, dried
3/4 cup	raisins
1 tsp	preserved ginger (more if desirable)
1 tbsp	honey
1 tbsp	fruit juice (apple or orange)
1 tbsp	LSA
1 cup	coconut, toasted

Mince dried fruit and ginger
Combine in a bowl with honey, fruit juice, LSA and 1/2 of the coconut. Mix well
Form mixture into small balls and roll in the remaining coconut
Slightly flatten to form thick button shapes
Refrigerate until firm then store in fridge in an airtight container
Can be made several days ahead

Rhubarb

This is tasty served with soy custard or baked bread custard

500gm	fresh rhubarb, washed trimmed and cut into pieces
2 cups	water
½ tsp	white stevia powder
1	fresh banana

Cover rhubarb with water, add stevia powder and slowly bring to the boil
Simmer for 2 to 3 minutes
Remove from heat, cool, then add sliced banana
Serve with muesli for breakfast, or with soy custard for dessert

Fruity petit fours

1 cup	dried pears, chopped
1/2 cup	dried apricots, chopped
1/2 cup	cashews, chopped
1/2 cup	shredded coconut
1 tbsp	lemon juice
1 pinch	white stevia powder
425ml/15oz	coconut cream

Mix all ingredients together with enough coconut cream to bind the

mixture
Stand covered for 1 hour
If mixture is too dry, add more coconut cream to hold it together and make it pliable
Roll into small balls. Press a cashew nut into top of each ball
Place in small confectionery paper-patty cups
Cover and store in fridge in an airtight container

Peachy treats

Made in a flash, this dessert is light and very tasty
Peach or pear halves can be used

825g/30oz	peach halves, drained or 6 - 8 fresh peaches
100g/3-4oz	natural soy yoghurt
1 cup	mixed dried fruit, chopped
1 tbsp	apple or orange juice
1 pinch	ground cinnamon
1/2 cup	toasted coconut

Arrange peach halves in individual serving dishes
Mix fruit juice with dried fruit
Stand for about 1/2 hour, then fold into yoghurt
Spoon mixture into hollows of peaches, sprinkle with cinnamon
Top each serve with coconut
Serves 6 to 8

Baked bread custard

4	large eggs
3 cups	soy milk
1 level tsp	stevia powder
1/2 cup	coconut
2 to 3	slices fruit-loaf or wholemeal bread
1 tbsp	natural sultanas
½ tsp	vanilla essence
½ tsp	ground nutmeg or cinnamon

Cut bread into pieces
Place in a 2 litre/70oz capacity ovenproof dish and sprinkle with sultanas
Beat eggs with stevia, stir in milk, vanilla and coconut, pour over fruit loaf or bread and sprinkle with spices
Place dish in a baking pan with about 2.5cm (1 inch) of hot water
Bake at 160°C/300F and bake for around 1 hour until custard is set
Serves 6

Fruits and flakes biscuits

Store in airtight container.

5 cups	cornflakes or riceflakes
1 cup	coconut
1/4 cup	flaxseeds, ground
¼ tsp	white stevia powder
1 cup	natural sultanas
1 cup	dates, chopped
1 cup	wholemeal SR flour
3/4 cup	cold pressed olive oil
2	eggs, lightly beaten

Combine all dry ingredients in a large bowl, add oil and eggs
Mix well
Take heaped dessertspoons of mixture, mould into round shapes
Press lightly with hand
Place on an oiled oven tray about 2.5cm (1 inch) apart
Bake in a moderate oven for about 10 minutes until golden brown
Leave on tray for a few minutes
Place on a wire rack to cool

Chocolate fruit loaf

No eggs, sugar or fat

1 cup	mixed dried fruit
1 level tsp	white stevia powder
1 cup	wheatgerm or oat bran
1and 1/2 cups	oat, soy or rice milk
1/4 cup	cocoa powder
1 cup	wholemeal SR flour

Place fruits, wheat germ (or oat bran) and milk in a large bowl
Cover and let stand for 2 hours
Fold in sifted cocoa and flour and mix well
Place in loaf tin lined with baking paper and bake at 160°C for 30 mins, then test with a skewer, if still uncooked, bake for a further 10 mins
Cool in tin for 5 mins, turn out onto rack in a tea towel to keep moist until cooled
Store in airtight tin

Tangy fruit loaf

1/4 cup	cold pressed oil
¼ cup	brown sugar and ¼ to ½ tsp white stevia powder
1	egg
3	bananas, sliced

½ cup	dates, chopped
1and ½ cups	wholemeal SR flour
½ cup	wheatgerm
½ tsp	bi-carb soda
½ cup	pecan, brazil or walnuts, chopped
1tbsp	lemon, juice

Warm oil and sugar in saucepan and stir until sugar dissolves. Cool
Add egg and beat well, stir in bananas, dates, nuts and lemon juice
Add sifted flour, wheatgerm and soda
Fold in and blend well
Pour into greased loaf tin
Bake in a moderate oven for about 1 hour

Banana cake

250g/9oz	wholemeal SR flour
½ cup	cold pressed oil
70g	raw sugar and ½ tsp white stevia powder
2 large	ripe bananas, mashed
3 tbsp	soy or rice milk
1 tsp	bi-carb soda
1 tsp	vanilla
2	eggs

Beat oil and sugar until smooth, add stevia and eggs, beat well
Add mashed bananas, mix milk, soda and vanilla together
Add alternately with sifted flour until all ingredients are folded smoothly together
Place mixture in a lined cake tin
Sprinkled with cinnamon or chopped walnuts
Cook in a moderate oven for about 45 minutes, test with skewer
Cool in tin for 10 minutes before removing to a cooling rack

Poached fruitee pears

3	large pears, peeled and cored
1/2 cup	dried apricots, chopped
1/2 cup	shredded coconut
1/4 cup	almonds, chopped
1/2 tsp	cinnamon
1 tsp	honey (more if desired)
1 cup	apple or apricot juice

Cut pears in half and lay centre-up in a casserole dish
In a bowl mix together apricots, coconut, almonds and cinnamon
Add enough honey to bind the mixture together

Divide the mixture evenly over the six pear halves
Add one cup of juice to casserole, pour gently over the fruit
Cover and bake in preheated oven at 180°C/350°F, approx 30 minutes
Serve barely warm, with apple and pear ice cream, or next best cream
Serves 4 or more

Apple and Pear ice cream

1	pear, stem removed, skin on
1	granny smith apple, skin on
1/2 cup	soy milk
1 tsp	honey or 2 pinches stevia powder
1 small scoop	soy yoghurt
1 tbsp	gelatine, or agar agar
425ml/15oz	coconut milk

Mix all ingredients together in a food processor or blender, until smooth
Pour into a container of your choice and freeze
Serve in scoops with crushed almonds or with poached pears
Serves 4

Dried Pear Delights

500g	dried pears minced
2 tsp	powdered ginger
2 tsp	powdered cinnamon
1/2 cup	fresh lemon juice
250 g	smooth nut spread (such as ABC Melrose)
1/2 cup	dessicated coconut

Whole almonds or cashews
Mix all ingredients together, except whole nuts, until well combined and firm.
Take a whole nut and cover with mixture, and roll into a ball. Can use extra coconut, when rolling, if mixture is sticky.
Repeat until all mixture is used. Store in airtight container in fridge. Will keep for months if frozen.
Note: Lovers of ginger may use minced preserved ginger for stronger flavour.
Option: Substitute dried apricots with fresh orange juice for variety.

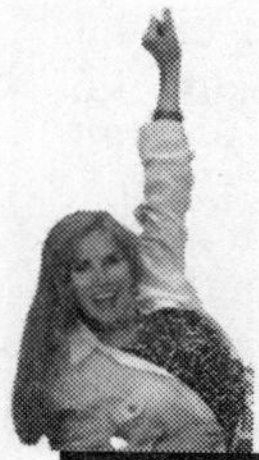

Farewell Message
Aurevoir or bye for now

I do hope that you have enjoyed reading this book and that it has put the missing pieces of the jigsaw puzzle back together for you.

Writing this book has been a long journey for me. I wanted to write this book two years ago, but I needed time to do more research. This book is the culmination of talking to thousands of overweight people face to face, by e-mail, in seminars, in health food stores and in my clinic. I have surfed the infinite web of the Internet for innumerable hours, questioned many experts, and read many books on the subject of metabolism and Syndrome X. I agreed with some of their theories, but in most books I found that the recipes did not match up with the theory. What's more there was incredible divergence of opinion amongst the so-called experts. Some believed that the process of rapid fat burning, which leads to ketosis, was dangerous, whereas others thought it was the pathway to the Holy Grail of slimness. Some worshipped low - fat high - carbohydrate diets, some worshipped high - fat high - protein diets and some worshipped low - carbohydrate high - protein diets. If you had time to read all of these books, you would have a huge theoretical knowledge, but would probably be very confused.

As usual I found that none of these books considered the liver as vitally important in the genesis of obesity. This oversight has always been astonishing to me, especially as today we are seeing an epidemic of fatty livers.

Amusingly I found that many of the experts were critical of each other's theories and books, but all held their own grains of truth amongst the confusion.

As always in life you come to the conclusion that you must tell your story the way you see it and understand it, in your own unique style. So I have tried to separate the wheat from the chaff, and present a balanced hybrid of modern day research and opinion, coloured with my own clinical experience.

Most of you will have tried many different diets with varied success, but how many of you are feeling that you are looking and feeling the best you can possibly be? According to current statistics not many of us!

Between 1980 and 1995 the average Australian woman put on 4.8 kilograms and the average Australian male put on an extra 3.6 kilograms. Between 1980 and 2000 the number of women between 25 and 64 years of age who were overweight, increased from 27% to 45%. That's a big increase!

More than half of adult Australians are overweight and 19% of these are obese. This means that approximately 7.5 million Australians are battling with their weight.

Sixty four percent of men and 49% of women are overweight or obese.

Australians tend to get fatter with increasing age – approximately 38% of men aged between 19 and 24 are overweight or obese, and 75% of men aged between 45 to 64 are overweight. Comparable statistics for women are 26% aged between 19 and 24, and 60% aged between 45 to 64.

It is obvious that weight excess becomes far more common as we become older.

This can be explained by the following factors –

- Liver dysfunction and fatty liver become more common with age, especially in our modern day environment.
- The chemical imbalance of Syndrome X becomes more pronounced as we age, especially with the modern day refined high carbohydrate diet.
- Our hormones tend to wear out before we do, resulting in a slowing down of metabolism with age.
- We are inclined to exercise less, as we become more involved in family and business activities and neglect ourselves.

It could be said that we become "middle-aged" when our age starts to show around our middle. The term "middle-aged spread" is a well-known saying, and has come to be accepted as almost inevitable.

This book has been written to tell you that you do not have to accept these things as inevitable. No one wants to become overweight and unhealthy just because they are 45. Hell, that is when life begins!

Young people are also increasingly suffering with obesity, and the average age of onset of "mature aged diabetes" is getting younger.

You do not have to be part of these statistics! You now have the knowledge, and thus the ability, to overcome the hormonal and metabolic problems that have been causing you to get fatter and fatter. It's really not that hard if you use my strategic plan. This plan attacks successfully all the causes that are keeping you trapped in the chemical imbalances, which lead to excess weight.

Stay in touch...
DR SANDRA CABOT WEIGHT LOSS CLINICS

I have trained a network of consultants in Australia who can help you to implement the Syndrome X eating plan into your life.
This is because -

- You may need help to plan your own recipes and make the changes in your diet and lifestyle that it will take to achieve your goals.
- You may suffer with food allergies or intestinal complaints that make it necessary to modify this eating program slightly.
- You may be confused about your Body Type.
- You may be confused about the concept of Syndrome X and if this chemical imbalance is really affecting you to a major degree.
- You may need to be put in touch with a doctor in your city who understands the use of natural hormone creams and lozenges.
- You may be a very busy person who would like to have your meals delivered to your door, so you are not tempted to indulge in unhealthy sugary foods.
- You may need someone who is truly interested in your outcome and will work with you and monitor your progress and make the necessary adjustments to your program over time.
- You may need to speak with someone who has experienced the wonderful life changing experience of balancing their metabolism, which can only be achieved by correcting all the factors that are keeping you fat.
- You may need inspiring, you may need encouragement and you may just need someone to hold your hand.

Whatever it takes, we promise to help you achieve your goals!

To be put in touch with one of the Dr Sandra Cabot Weight Loss Consultants call 02 4655 8855. We are there to help you – don't be shy – pick up the phone now and change your life today!

REFERENCES

Ref. 1. Reaven GM Pathophysiology of insulin resistance in human disease. Physiological Reviews. 1995;75(3):473-485.

Ref. 2. Assmann G, Schulte H. The importance of triglycerides: results from the Prospective Cardiovascular Muenster (PROCAM) Study. Eur J Epidemiol 1992; Supplement 1:99-103;Assmann G.Schulte H. Relation of high-density lipoprotein cholesterol and triglycerides to incidence of atherosclerotic coronary artery disease (the PROCAM experience). Am J Cardiology 1992; 70:733-37.

Ref. 3. Reissell P K et al. Treatment of hypertriglyceridaemia. Am J Clin Nutr 1966; 19:84 - 98.

Ref. 4. Sanchez - Delgado E, Liechti H. Lifetime risk of developing coronary heart disease. Lancet 1999; 353:934.

Ref. 5. U.S. Bureau of Census.

Ref. 6. Smith M A et al. Advanced Maillard reaction end products are associated with Alzheimer disease pathology. Proc Nat Acad Sci USA 1994; 91:5710 - 14 and Vitek M P et al. Advanced glycation end products contribute to amyloidosis in Alzheimer disease Proc Nat Acad Sci USA 1994; 91: 4766 - 70.

Ref. 7. - Gymnema Sylvestre

Use of Gymnema Sylvestre Leaf Extract in the control of blood glucose in insulin-dependent diabetes mellitus, Shanmugasundaram. G et al. Dept. Biochemistry, University of Madras, Madras 600-113, Elsevier Scientific Publishers Ireland 1990

Studies on the Hypoglycaemic Action of Gymnema Sylvestre, Dept. Biochemistry, University of Madras 600 042, Arogya -J. Health Sci., 1981, VII, 38-60.

Antidiabetic Effect of a leaf extract from Gymnema Sylvestre in non-insulin dependent diabetes mellitus patients, K. Baskaran et al. Journal of Ethnopharmacology, 30(1990) 295-305, Elsevier Scientific Publishers Ireland Ltd.

Ref. 8. - Momordica charantia (Bitter Melon)

Leatherdale, B.A. et al. Improvement in glucose tolerance due to Momordica charantia, (1981) British Medical Journal, 282: 1823-1824.

Sarkar, S. et al. Demonstration of the hypoglycaemic action of Momordica charantia in a validated animal model of diabetes. 1996

Pharmacological Research, 33(1):1-4.
Akhtar M.S. (1982) Trial of Momordica charantia powder in patients with maturity onset diabetes. Journal of the Pakistan Medical Association. 32:106-107
Welihinda, J. et al. Effect of Momordica charantia on the glucose tolerance in maturity onset diabetes.1986, J. Ethnopharmacology 17:277-282
Cunnick J. 1993, Bitter Melon, Journal of Naturopathic Medicine. 4(1): 261

Ref. 9 & 10. - Chromium
Kaats GR et al. Effects of chromium picolinate on body composition. A randomised double-masked, placebo-controlled study. Current Therap. Research (1996) 57(10):747-765
Anderson RA et al. Elevated intakes of supplemental chromium improve glucose and insulin variables in individuals with type II diabetes. Diabetes (1997);46:1786-91
Cunningham JJ. Micronutrients as nutraceutical interventions in diabetes mellitus. J. Am Coll Nutr. 1998;17(1):7-10

Ref. 11. - Lipoic Acid
Sachse G & Willms B. Efficiency of thioctic acid (lipoic acid) in the therapy of peripheral diabetic neuropathy. Hormone & Metabolic Research (Supplement). 9:105, 1980
Wagh SS et al. Mode of action of lipoic acid in diabetes. Journal of Bioscience. 11:59-74, 1987.
Chromium Picolinate
Liu, V. J., Chromium & Insulin in young subjects with normal glucose tolerance. Am. J. Clin. Nutr. 25(4) 1982, pp. 661-667
Jacob S. et al. Enhancement of glucose disposal in patients with type 2 diabetes by alpha-lipoic acid. Arzneim - Rorsch Drug Res. 1995;45(2):872-874
Jacob S. et al. The antioxidant alpha-lipoic acid enhances insulin-stimulated glucose metabolism in insulin-resistant rat skeletal muscle. Diabetes. 1996;45:1024-1029
Jacobs et al. Enhancement of glucose disposal in patients with type 11 diabetes by alpha-lipoic acid. Arzneimittel-Forschung (1993) 45:872-74
Strodter D et al. The influence of lipoic acid (thioctic acid) on metabolism and function of the diabetic heart. Diabetic Res. Clin. Prac. (1995) 29(1):19-26
Packer L et al. Neuro protection by the metabolic antioxidant alpha

lipoic acid. Free Radical Biol. Med. (1997) 22(1-2): 359-78

Khamaisis M: Lipoic acid reduces glycaemia and increases muscle GLUT 4 content in diabetic rats. Metabolism 46(7), 763-768 (1997)

Jacob S; The antioxidant alpha-lipoic acid enhances insulin-stimulated glucose metabolism in insulin-resistant rat skeletal muscle. Diabetes 45(8), 1024-1029 (1996)

Ziegler D et al. (1997) Alpha-lipoic acid in the treatment of diabetic peripheral and cardiac autonomic neuropathy. Diabetes 46 (Suppl 2): S62-S66

Ref. 12. - Carnitine

Opie LH. Role of carnitine in fatty acid metabolism of normal & ischaemic myocardium Am. Heart J. 97:375-388, 1979

Pola P. et al. Carnitine in the therapy of dyslipidaemic patients. Curr. Ther. Res. 27:208 - 216, 1980

Rebouche CJ and Engel AG. Carnitine metabolism & Deficiency Syndromes. Mayo Clinic Proceedings. 58:533 - 540, 1983

Rossi CS & Siliprandi N. Effect of carnitine on serum HDL-cholesterol: report of cases. John Hopkins Medical Journal. 150:51-54, 1982

Sachan DS et al. Ameliorating effect of carnitine & its precursors on alcohol-induced fatty liver. Am. J. Clin. Nutr. 39:738-744, 1984

Ref. 13. - Selenium

Margaret Rayman, "Dietary Selenium; time to act", British Medical Journal, Vol. 314, 387, Feb 1997

Ref. 14. - Zinc

Solomon, S.J. et al, Effect of low zinc intake on carbohydrate & fat metabolism in men. Federal Proc. 42 (1983), p.391.

Tauri, S. Studies of zinc metabolism: Effect of the diabetic state on zinc metabolism: A clinical aspect. Endocrinology Japan 10 (1963), pp. 9-15

Faure P. et al. Zinc prevents the structural and functional properties of free radical treated-insulin. Biochimica et Biophysica Acta. 1994;1209:260-264

Ref. 15. - Silymarin (St Mary's Thistle)

Boari C, et al, Occupational toxic liver diseases. Therapeutic effects of Silymarin. Min Med 1985; 72(2):679-88

Valenzuela A. et al. Silybin protects rat erythrocytes against phenylhydrazine-induced lipid peroxidation and haemolysis. Planta Medica. 53:402-405, 1987

Vengerovski AI et al. Liver protective action of silybinene in experimental CCL4 poisoning. Farmakologiya Toksikologiya. 50:67-

69, 1987

Wagner H. Antihepatoxic flavonoids. Progress in Clinical and Biological Research. 213:319-331, 1986

Flora K, et al. Milk Thistle (Silybum marianum) for the therapy of liver disease. Am. J. Gastroenterol 1998 Feb; 93(2): 139-43

Salmi HA, et al, Effect of silymarin on chemical, functional and morphological alteration of the liver: a double blind controlled study. Scandinavian J. Gastroenterology 1982; 17:417-21

Valenzuela A. et al. Silymarin protection against hepatic lipid peroxidation. Biochemical Pharmacology 34:2209-2212, 1985

Floersheim GL.et al. Effects of penicillin & silymarin on liver enzymes and blood clotting factors in dogs given a boiled preparation of Amanita Phalloides. Toxicology & Applied Pharmacology. 46:455-462, 1978

Vogel G. A peculiarity among the flavonoids: silymarin, a compound active on the liver. Munich Proceedings of the International Bioflavonoid Symposium. 461-480, 1981

Valenzueal A. et al. Silymarin protection against hepatic lipid peroxidation induced by acute ethanol intoxication in the rat. Biochemical Pharmacology. 34:2209-2212, 1985

Ref. 16. - Taurine

Orthoplex Research Bulletin, Taurine the detoxifying amino acid. Nutrients in profile, Henry Osiecki. Bioconcepts Publishing

Ref. 17. - Globe Artichoke

S. Rocchietta, Minerva Med. 50, 612, 1959)

Liver Function

Parveen J. Kumar BSc. MD, FRCP, Clinical Medicine, Liver Function, page 237-287, Bailliere Tindall

Ref. 18. - Von Herbay A et al. Vitamin E improves the aminotransferase status of patients suffering with viral hepatitis C: a randomised, double-blind, placebo-controlled trial. Free Radical Res 1997 Dec;27(6):599-605

Ref. 19. - Bland J.S., Bralley J.A. Nutritional up-regulation of hepatic detoxification enzymes. The Journal of Applied Nutrition, 1992,44; No. 3 & 4

Cabre E, et al. Nutritional Support in liver disease. Eur J Gastroenterol Hepatol 1995;7(6): 528-32

Meister A. Selective modification of glutathione metabolism. Science 220:472-477, 1983, The Doctor's Vitamin Encyclopedia, Arrow

Books, Dr Sheldon Hendler. M.D., PhD.
Professor Robin Fraser, Lipoproteins & the Liver Sieve. Hepatology 21:863-874. 1995
Diseases of the Liver & Biliary System, Dr Sheila Sherlock, Blackwell Press
Nutritional Influences on Illness, A Source Book of Clinical Research, Melvyn R. Werbach. MD
The Doctor's Vitamin Encyclopedia, Dr Sheldon Hendler, MD., PhD.
Leiber CS, et al. Role of dietary adipose & endogenously synthesised fatty acids in the pathogenesis of the alcoholic fatty liver. J. Clin Invest 1966; 45:51-62

Statin Drugs

Ref. 20. Journal of the American Medical Association (1996; 275:55-60),

Ref. 21. Nature Medicine, December, 2000; 6:1311-1312, 1399-1402

Ref. 22. Psychosomatic Medicine 2000; 62.

Stevia

Jeppesen PB, et al. Stevioside acts directly on pancreatic beta cells to secrete insulin. Metabolism 2000 Feb;49(2):208-14
Akashi, J. and Yokohama. Safety of extract of dried stevia leaves - results of toxicity tests. Shokuhin Kogya, 10B:34-43, 1975
Bridel M. and Lavielle. Le principe a saveur sucree du Kaa-he-e (Stevia rebaudiana Bertoni). J. Pharm. Clin, 14:99-154, 1931
Kinghorn A.D. et al. Current status of stevioside as a sweetening agent for human use. Economic and Medicinal Plant Research, London: Academic Press, Inc., 1985
Ishii- Iwamoto et al. Stevioside is not metabolised in the isolated perfused rat liver. Research Communications in Molecular Pathology & Pharmacology, 87:167-175, 1995
Crammer B. and R. Ikan, Progress in the chemistry and properties of stevia rebaudioside. Developments in Sweeteners. London, Elsevier, vol. 3:45-64, 1987
Fletcher, Hewitt, Jr. The sweet herb of Paraguay. Chemurgic Digest, 18, July/August, 1955

Aspartame

Olney J. W., N.B. Farber et al. Increasing brain tumour rates: is there a link to aspartame? Journal of Neuropathology & Experimental Neurology, 55(11):1115-1123, 1996

Ref. 23. Suttajit M. et al. Mutagenicity and human chromosomal effects of stevioside, a sweetener from stevia rebaudiana. Environmental Health Perspectives Supplement, 101 (3):53-56, 1993.
Pezzuto, J.M. et al. Metabolically activated steviol, the aglycone of stevioside is mutagenic. Proceedings of the National Academy of Sciences, 82(8): 2478-2482, 1985

Ref. 24 & 25. Curi, R., M. Alvarez, et al. Effect of stevia rebaudiana on glucose tolerance in normal adult humans. Brazilian Journal of Medicine & Biological Research, 19(6):771-774, 1986 and Alvarez M. et al. Effect of aqueous extract of stevia rebaudiani on biochemical parameters of normal adult persons. Arq. Biol. Tech, 24:178, 1981
Nunes, P., and N.A. Pereira. The effect of stevia rebaudiana on the fertility of experimental animals. Revista Brasileira de Farmacia, 69:46-50, 1988
Klongpanichpak, S., et al. lack of mutagenicity of stevioside and steviol in Salmonella typhimurium TA 98 & TA 100. Journal Medical Associations of Thailand, Sep; 80, Suppl 1:S121-128, 1997

Ref. 26. Melis, M.S. A crude extract of Stevia rebaudiana increases the renal plasma flow of normal and hypertensive rats. Brazilian Journal of Medicine & Biological Research, 29(5):660-675, 1996
Yodyingyaud, V. et al. Effect of Stevioside on growth and reproduction. Human Reproduction, 6(1):158-165, 1991
Toyada K. et al. Assessment of the carcinogenicity of stevioside in F344 rats. Food & Chemical Toxicology, 35(6):597-603, 1997
Xili, L. et al. Chronic oral toxicity and carcinogenicity study of stevioside in rats. Food Chemistry Toxicology, 30:957-965, 1992
Von Schmelling, G.A., et al. Stevia rebaudiani : Evaluation of the hypoglycaemic effect in alloxanized rabbits. Ciencia e Cultura, 29(5):599-601, 1977

Ref. 27. D L Tirshwell, Presentation 24th Annual AHA Conference on Stroke and Cerebral Circulation Feb 10th 1999

Ref. 28. Dreon D M, Fernstrom H A, Williams P T, Krauss R M. A very low-fat diet is not associated with improved lipoprotein profiles in men with a predominance of large, low-density lipoproteins. Am J Clin Nutr 1999; 69:411-18

Ref. 29. Albert C M et al. Fish consumption and risk of sudden cardiac death. JAMA 1998; 279:23-28.

Ref. 30. Barnard D E et al. Dietary transfatty acids modulate erythrocyte membrane fatty acyl composition and insulin binding in monkeys. J Nutr Biochem 1990; 1:190-95; Kuller L H. Transfatty acids and dieting (letter). Lancet 1993; 341:1093-94
Mann G V. Metabolic consequences of dietary transfatty acids. Lancet 1994; 343:1268-71

Ref. 31.
Willett W C, et al. Intake of transfatty acids of risk of coronary heart disease among women. Lancet 1993; 341:581-85

Ref. 32.
Glutamine
Ballard T. et al. Effect of Glutamine Supplementation on impaired glucose regulation during intravenous lipid administration. Dept. of Surgery, Duke University Medical Centre and Veterans Affairs Medical Centre, Durham, North Carolina, USA. Nutrition 1996;12:349-354

Ref. 33.
Glucagon
Muller, W. A. et al. The Influence of the antecedent diet upon glucagon and insulin secretion. New England Journal of Medicine 285 (1971), pp. 1450 - 1454.

Diabetes

Reaven P. Dietary & pharmacological regimes to reduce lipid peroxidation in non-insulin-dependent diabetes mellitus. Am. J. Clin. Nutr. 1995;62:1483S-1489S

Thompson KH. Et al. Micronutrients and antioxidants in the progression of diabetes. Nutrition Research 1995;15(9):1377-1410
Schleicher E. et al. Increased accumulation of the glycoxidation product N (epsilon) - (carboxymethyl) lysien in human tissues in diabetes and ageing. Journal of Clinical Investigations, 99:457-468, 1997

FemmePhase™

CHC 30703-01/03

FemmePhase has been known to Australian women as a high quality nutritional supplement for several years.

FemmePhase has now been improved to provide -

- A much higher dose of calcium
- A standardised amount of isoflavones (phyto-estrogens) equivalent to a daily dose of 40mg isoflavone glycosides.

FemmePhase is indicated for:

- The maintenance of general health and wellbeing of pre-menopausal and post-menopausal women
- The relief of the symptoms of menopause including hot flushes.

FemmePhase contains 2 different types of calcium, as women's calcium requirements are increased by menopause. Calcium supplementation may be of assistance in the prevention of osteoporosis. **FemmePhase** is packed with ***minerals***, ***vitamins*** and ***herbs*** to provide you with a comprehensive formula, which means that you do not have to take a lot of different tablets.

Comparison of Popular over the counter products*

How they compare	Menopause	Phytolife	Remifemin	Promensil	FemmePhase
Red Leaf Clover					50mg/day
Isoflavones (Red Clover)				40mg/day	
Black Cohosh	500mg/day		104mg/day		50mg/day
Soy isoflavones	60mg/day	64mg/day			40mg/day
Dong Quai					50mg/day
Wild yam					860mg/day
Liquorice root					50mg/day
Kelp					50mg/day
Horsetail					50mg/day
Sarsparilla					50mg/day
Alfalfa					50mg/day
Calcium	80mg/day	668mg/day			505mg/day
Magnesium	40mg/day				10mg/day
Zinc					400mcg/day
Added vitamins	YES	NO	NO	NO	YES
Bioflavonoids	NO	NO	NO	NO	YES

*All quantities are as supplied on corresponding product label and calculated on the recommended daily basis. Non standardised herbs are calculated on an equivalent to dry herb basis.

FemmePhase is available in all good health food stores and pharmacies

Are You Running Out of Steam?

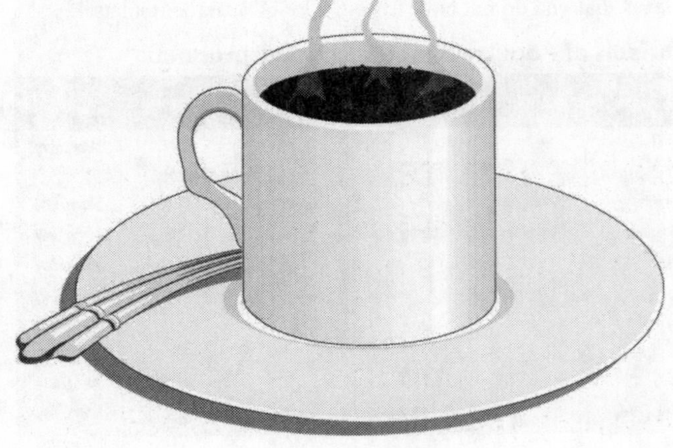

If so
Your Hormones may need Balancing

The Sandra Cabot Hormone Balancing & Weight Control Clinic

WE SPECIALISE IN:

1. Natural Hormone Replacement using state of the art hormonal creams and lozenges. Every woman is individually assessed with the aim of fine-tuning.
2. Hormonal imbalances
3. Weight control using the techniques in this book
4. Body Shaping counselling
5. Nutritional advice and natural therapies

OUR EXPERT TEAM CONSISTS OF:

Medical Doctors

Naturopaths and Nutritionists

For appointments
phone (02) 4655 8855 or (02) 9328 2900

Sandra Cabot Health Clinic

33

285 Ne ... ff

(near Rail ... ir)

G.K. Products, Inc.
10088 N.W. 3rd Place
Coral Springs, Fl 33071
1-888-752-4286

Conversion Chart for Recipes and Cooking

Ounces	Grams
1	28
2	57
3	85
4	113
5	142
6	170
7	198
8	227
9	255
10	283

For additional amounts select the appropriate conversion above, and multiply, or add, or both.
For example 15 ounces = 10 ounces (283 grams)
+5 ounces (142 grams) = 15 ounces (425 grams)

Pounds	Kilograms
1	0.45
2	0.91
3	1.36
4	1.81
5	2.27
6	2.72
7	3.17
8	3.63
9	4.10
10	4.54

Farenheit (°F)	Centigrade (°C)
200	93
250	121
300	149
350	177
400	204

For other temperature conversions use the following formula:
F to C: subtract 32, then divide by 1.8
C to F: multiply by 1.8, then add 32.

Kitchen Measures

Measure	Ounces	Millilitres
One teaspoon	0.17	5
One tablespoon	0.5	14
One cup	8	227
One pint	16	454
One quart	32	908
One gallon	128	3632

Helpful Conversion Chart

Ounces to millilitres:
multiply ounce figure by 30 to get number of millilitres

Pounds to Kilograms:
multiply pound figure by 0.45 to get number of kilograms

Pounds to grams:
multiply pound figure by 453 to get number of grams

Grams to ounces:
multiply gram figure by 0.0353 to get number of ounces

Ounces to grams:
multiply ounce figure by 28.3 to get number of grams

One teaspoon = 5 grams
Three teaspoons = one tablespoon = 1/2 ounce = 14.3 grams
Two tablespoons = one ounce = 28.35 grams
Agar-agar (1 bar) = 4-6 tablespoons agar-agar flakes
Garlic concentrate (1 teaspoon) - 2 cloves fresh garlic.
Herbs, dried (1/4 teaspoon) = 2 tablespoons fresh herbs.

Sweeteners Equivalents

1/2 cup sweetener =	1/2 cup maple syrup
	1/2 cup coconut sugar
	1/2 cup raw sugar
	1/3 cup molasses
	1/2 cup honey
	1+1/2 cups barley malt extract
	1/2 cup fruit juice concentrate
	1/2 cup fruit juice
	1/2 cup unsweetened frozen juice concentrate